CLINICAL COMPANION

Van Leuven

FUNDAMENTALS OF NURSING

SIXTH EDITION

**Kozier • Erb
Berman • Burke**

Prentice Hall Health
Upper Saddle River, New Jersey 07458

Project Editors: Virginia Simione Jutson, Grace Wong
Managing Editor: Wendy Earl
Associate Editor: Stephanie Kellogg
Publishing Assistants: Susan Teahan, Peggy Hammett
Production Supervisor: David Novak
Production Coordination: Sondra Kirkley Glider
Interior Design: The Left Coast Group, Inc
Cover Design: Yvo Riezebos Design
Typesetting: The Left Coast Group, Inc.
Printer/Binder: Banta
Cover Illustration: The quilt is entitled *Summer's End*,
© Joy Saville. Photo by William Taylor.
Director of Manufacturing and Production: Bruce Johnson
Manufacturing Buyer: Ilene Sanford

Previously published by Addison-Wesley Nursing
A Division of the Benjamin/Cummings Publishing
Company, Inc.
Redwood City, California 94065

10 9 8 7 6 5 4 3 2

ISBN 0–8053–8353–0

Prentice-Hall International (UK) Limited, London
Prentice-Hall of Australia Pty. Limited, Sydney
Prentice-Hall Canada Inc., Toronto
Prentice-Hall Hispanoamericana, S.A., Mexico
Prentice-Hall of India Private Limited, New Delhi
Prentice-Hall of Japan, Inc., Tokyo

CLINICAL COMPANION

Karen Van Leuven, RN, PhD
Samuel Merritt College
Oakland, California

Western University of Health Sciences
Pomona, California

FOREWORD

The *Clinical Companion* for *Fundamentals of Nursing* has been created to serve as a resource for students in the clinical area. It provides succinct information to guide you as you begin this important, exciting, and challenging component of your nursing program. Much of the content has been suggested by nursing students we consulted during the book's planning stages.

To keep this practical guide compact and portable, we have summarized key information designed to reinforce content that first must be learned thoroughly and carefully from the text, *Fundamentals of Nursing*. The *Clinical Companion* is not intended in any way to replace the text; rather, its purpose is to help you recall key points as you prepare to deliver safe and effective nursing care in a dynamic clinical environment. Before proceeding with the suggested guidelines and actions given in this book, check to determine an agency's policies, practices, and protocol.

The *Clinical Companion* opens with a Quick Reference unit that presents essential information you'll be able to retrieve rapidly. Subsequent units, organized according to the steps of the nursing process, provide summaries to address the clinically related topics you can expect to encounter routinely. Finally, we provide an index that will guide you quickly to the information you need. As you gain expertise in the clinical area, we believe you'll continue to consult the *Clinical Companion* again and again.

PREFACE

Welcome to the nursing profession! You are embarking on a career that offers many challenges and rewards. As a faculty member, a clinical instructor, and a colleague, I would like to share with you some tips that may help you in your transition to professional nursing.

Nursing education, and clinical education in particular, can be very challenging and stressful. Often, students know the right answers, but are too nervous to think or to articulate their thoughts. Hence, my first words of wisdom: Relax! Also, never be afraid to let your instructors know what you don't know. Your instructors can't help you unless you make them aware of your need for direction. Good nurses are those who know what they don't know and who know when to seek advice or counsel.

Nursing can be a humbling profession. Like all nurses, I am constantly reminded of how much I don't know. New drugs appear regularly, as do advances in treatments and protocols. To ensure that you provide safe nursing care, therefore, you need to practice within your scope of knowledge and experience. Asking for assistance also invites discussion and collaboration.

There are many ways to accomplish a given task; therefore, be accepting of different ways of practice. The right way to practice nursing care is simply the way that is safe and that works for you and the client. As you watch others perform skills, ask yourself whether the goals were met and the care was safe. If these criteria are met, then good nursing care was delivered. Many novice nurses are disappointed when they see another nurse practice in a way different from what they have learned. In some instances, a difference may represent real problems; in others, it may simply be a different style of delivering safe nursing care.

Watch other nurses and learn from them. Look for positive role models. Take advantage of your learning experience, and seek exposure to different clients. Offer to help other students and staff so you can be part of the team. Read about how to practice nursing. Practice your skills in the laboratory to foster confidence. But, above all, become involved with nursing care—this is how you become a nurse.

It's easy to be overwhelmed by all that you must learn, but it's important to consider what you, the new student, can offer as well. As our newest colleagues, you bring to the profession vitality, enthusiasm, and inspiration. New students remind me and others of the excitement that learning brings and of the challenges and stimulation nursing practice provides.

New students also bring innovation to the clinical area. As a beginner, you may fret over becoming proficient in tasks and skills; it's easy to want to "get it right" and do what the experienced nurse does. Unfortunately, this haste to fit in stifles creativity. Your fresh outlook may provide new insights into improving the way things are done.

On a personal level, you contribute spark, vigor, and contagious enthusiasm to our profession; don't underestimate the value of that contribution. This is a time of "firsts": first client, first care plan, first injection, first birth, first death, even first dirty bedpan! Along with all these firsts you are being asked to determine how you will become part of the change that will shape and focus the health care of tomorrow. In this endeavor I wish you the best of luck and warmly welcome you into the profession of nursing.

Karen Van Leuven, RN, PhD

CONTENTS

Unit 4: Documentation and Evaluation

INTRODUCTION

On the first day of my pediatrics rotation, one of the children assigned to me was a six-year-old asthmatic who had been hospitalized several times for this problem. Walking into his room with my instructor, I put forth what I thought was an air of confidence, even though my heart was beating a mile a minute. After the introductions, my little client reached for my hand and, with a voice of authority, told me not to be nervous, because he would tell me what I was supposed to do. Even though I was a little embarrassed that my cover was blown by a six-year-old, I had to chuckle at being comforted by the client I was supposed to make comfortable. Welcome to the world of clinical rotations!

Clinical rotations give the student the opportunity to translate classroom theory and laboratory skills into action. This necessary and exciting part of nursing education, however, is often accompanied by feelings of apprehension and awkwardness. New situations heighten these feelings, as does the realization that you are still in transition between learning a skill and knowing how to use it efficiently. But by being organized, being an active learner, and by being good to yourself, you can use these feelings to challenge yourself and turn your clinical experiences into fun learning experiences.

Nursing is undergoing a wonderful evolution, and as a student, you bring to the process fresh views. The clients you will care for, the staff you will work with, and the facts you will learn about yourself will all help shape your views and turn you into the effective professional you want to be. No matter how difficult your day is, you should look on it as a learning experience. These difficult days give you precious knowledge that will make future days go easier. Listed below are tips to help you avoid some of the pitfalls that make the clinical experience unnecessarily stressful.

Organize

Clinical days always bring a little apprehension. Even as a senior, when the routines were familiar and the knowledge base was more solid, I still asked myself: "What will my instructor ask me? What emergencies will upset the schedule I set for myself? What if I oversleep and I'm late?"

To help combat this apprehension, I always reminded myself that there was nothing routine about client care, even though people talked about "hospital routines." There are only two predictable actions in nursing: (1) clients will be cared for, and (2) documentation must be done. Everything else is subject to change!

To maintain your cool, do your work efficiently, and feel satisfied at the end of the day, you must be organized, set priorities, and remain flexible. Even if nothing else in your life is organized, be organized in your approach to the clinical experience. Remember also that organization and the ability to set priorities are behaviors instructors look for and grade on. The following are suggestions to help you become better organized:

- Arrive early. Set your alarm clock so that you arrive at the clinical site at least 20 minutes early. This gives you time to review the charts for any changes in doctor's orders, any orders that may have expired, or any tests that require your client to leave the floor. Doing this applies even if you cared for the same client the day before. Building in extra time also helps you on days when traffic is heavy or when you hit the snooze button once too often. The clinical experience can be stressful, so manage the stressors that are self-induced.

- Make a worksheet for reviewing charts. Include the name of the client, room number, diagnosis, primary nurse, times to assess vital signs, times to administer medications, equipment needs, procedures, and a space for comments. By making a note of the equipment you need, you can minimize the number of trips to the supply room (eg, for dressing changes). Write in red all procedures or medications that are time sensitive. In addition to helping you organize your information, this also facilitates note writing and reporting to the primary nurse. On page 4 is an example of a completed worksheet. See page 8 for a blank sample worksheet you can use.

- Check the client's medications when you get to the unit. Don't take for granted that a client's medications will be on the unit. In fact, one of the most stressful situations you can face is to find yourself running late because of an

Client's Name/Rm # Diagnosis Primary RN	Vital Signs Blood Sugars	Medication Times	IV's Catheters I & O	Treatments Procedures	Comments
Manouka, Kay #323 DKA Ms. Wallace RN	V.S.-qs B.S. 8 am 67 12 pm BO	8 am √ 12 pm √ 2 pm Cl. refused	IV's-none Caths-none I&O-strict	none	O.J. Given at 8 am No insulin given this shift
Banks, Martin #325 PUD Ms. Davies RN	V.S. q4 B.S. n/a	10 am √ 12 pm √ 2 pm √	IV-D5½ NS#2125/hr CATH-Foley I&O-none	UGI at 11 am Heme all stools Hep Flush q	NPO Client asked for communion this pm (called)

intervening emergency, only to discover that the client's medications are not on the unit; meanwhile, your instructor is waiting for you to give the medications. By checking the chart, you can prepare yourself for this situation. If an order has expired, notify the primary nurse or the physician promptly, and note the fact on the chart. This shows your professionalism and, more important, gives you control of the situation.

- Attend report and/or talk to the primary nurse before you start. As a student, you must act as independently as possible in assessments and decision making; however, it's wise to talk to the primary nurse, who has ultimate responsibility for the client's care. In particular, find out whether there's anything special you should know about the client. For example, the primary nurse may tell you that the client doesn't eat breakfast until his wife arrives at 8:30 AM. If this is not written in the chart, you may get yourself into a conflict with the client and learn about his preference the hard way. Knowing the details ahead of time can make your day easier.

- Do an "eyeball assessment" of each client's room before you start your day. Introduce yourself to the client and then look at whatever equipment is in the room. (Don't examine the client; you'll do that when your day begins.) Is there an IV? Is it dated and timed? Is it about to run out? Is there a catheter? Is the client being tube-fed? You will go over this information in report, but having it beforehand can help make you a more active participant. **Do your own inspection of** the unit, noting where the emergency cart is located, how the supply room is organized and where the bathroom is.

On your first day in a new unit or hospital, you will get an orientation to the unit. After this orientation, do your own inspection and find out how the supply room is organized, for example, where the 4 × 4 gauzes, catheter setups, and so on, are located. Review fire exits and where emergency equipment such as the "code" cart and fire extinguishers are located. Also, find out where the staff bathroom is! When you get busy, it's nice to be able to save steps.

By staying organized and taking control of those things that you can, you minimize stress and develop good habits that will stay with you throughout your career.

Learn Beyond the Here and Now

Nursing practice is based on understanding how to integrate knowledge from many sources and how to translate theory and facts into action. Clinical rotations offer a wonderful opportunity to do this, but you need to keep in mind that you need to focus primarily on how to help the client, not on how to get a good grade. Sometimes, the pressure to perform well for a good grade gets in the way of the learning experience. But if you focus on the needs of your client, a good grade will follow. As a nursing student, you have many ways to learn about nursing while still placing highest priority on your client's needs. **Review all pathophysiology and nursing theory related to your client's diagnosis, no matter how confident you feel about your knowledge base. After reviewing the pathophysiology, jot down** the laboratory studies, procedures, and medications you would expect to find ordered on the chart.

Also jot down signs and symptoms you would expect to see in the client. Compare your list to what actually appears in the chart. Compare your physical assessment findings with what you put on your list. How do the lists differ? How are they the same? **Don't let your title, "nursing student," prevent you from being an active member of the health care team.**

Ask questions of and talk with your instructor, other nurses, and doctors. Remember, the only dumb question is the one not asked. **Read journal articles that relate to your clients' diagnoses.**

Almost all hospitals have a library with current journals. After you leave the unit, make it a point to look for a new article that pertains to at least one of your clients. Imagine the pleasure of being able to answer an instructor's question about a client's course of treatment with, "A study reported in the latest issue of *Nursing Research* found that . . . . " This not only makes a positive impression, but also helps you learn. Although it may be tough to fit into your schedule, reading journals should become a habit.

Take Care of Yourself

Above all else, be good to yourself by taking care of yourself. There is no way to give good patient care if you can't concentrate because you are hungry or frazzled. The following are suggestions for minimizing some of life's irritations that can interfere with the business of learning nursing:

- Have a good breakfast. It may sound trite, but given the unpredictability of the hospital day,

Client's Name/Rm # Diagnosis Primary RN	Vital Signs Blood Sugars	Medication Times	IV's Catheters I & O	Treatments Procedures	Comments

you can't always depend on having time for a break or for lunch.

- Get your things together the night before.

- If you drive, make sure the car has gas. There's nothing worse than realizing at 6 AM that you are on empty and all the gas stations are closed.

- Keep some raisins or your favorite energy booster in your pocket for a quick pick-up.

- If you're feeling harried, stop for a minute and take a deep breath or two.

- Don't ever be afraid to ask for help.

- Keep a sense of humor.

Like anything else, the process of learning nursing can be frightening at first. The idea of practicing on real clients can be disconcerting. However, with some forethought and assertiveness, you can make the process fun, challenging, and a source of wonderful anecdotes to tell for years to come.

Best wishes for a great career in nursing.

Merilyn D. Francis, BSN, RN
1994 Graduate, University of the District of Columbia

UNIT 1

Quick Reference

A. Standard Precautions for All Client Care
B. Components of the Nursing Process
C. Communication Guidelines
D. Common Abbreviations
E. Medical Terminology
F. Weight and Volume Conversions and Equivalents
G. Laboratory Values
H. Common Diagnostic Studies
I. Nursing Interventions for Endoscopic Examinations
J. Studies of the Gastrointestinal Tract
K. Studies of the Gallbladder and Bile Ducts
L. Radiographic Studies: Intravenous Pyelography, Angiography, Myelography
M. Key Information About Vitamins
N. Key Information About Minerals
O. Infection Control Strategies
P. Recommended Childhood Immunization Schedule—U.S
Q. Immunization for High-Risk Adults

11

A. STANDARD PRECAUTIONS FOR ALL CLIENT CARE

CDC (HICPAC) Isolation Precautions (1996: updated 1997)

The Hospital Infection Control Practices Advisory Committee (HICPAC) of the CDC presented new guidelines for isolation precautions in hospitals in 1996. These guidelines designate two tiers of precautions:

Tier 1: Standard Precautions
Tier 2: Transmission-Based Precautions

Standard Precautions

These precautions are used in the care of all hospitalized persons regardless of their diagnosis or possible infection status. They apply to blood, all body fluids, secretions, and excretions *except sweat* (whether or not blood is present or visible), nonintact skin, and mucous membranes.

Thus they combine the major features of UP (Universal Precautions) and BSI (Body Substance Isolation). Recommended practices for Standard Precautions are shown in the following table.

Transmission-Based Precautions

These precautions are used in addition to Standard Precautions for clients with known or suspected infection that are spread in one of three ways: by airborne or droplet transmission, or by contact. The three types of transmission-based precautions may be used alone or in combination, but always **in addition** to Standard Precautions. They encompass all the conditions or diseases previously listed in the category-specific or disease-specific classifications devleoped by the CDC in 1983.

Recommended Isolation Precautions in Hospitals
(HICPAC 1996, revised February 17, 1997)

Standard Precautions (Tier One)

- Designed for *all* clients in hospital.

- These precautions apply to (1) blood; (2) all body fluids, excretions, and secretions except sweat; (3) nonintact (broken) skin; and (4) mucous membranes.

- Designed to reduce risk of transmission of microorganisms from recognized and unrecognized sources.

1. Wash hands after contact with blood, body fluids, secretions, excretions, and contaminated objects whether or not gloves are worn.

    a. Wash hands immediately after removing gloves.

    b. Use a nonantimicrobial soap for routine handwashing.

    c. Use an antimicrobial agent or an antiseptic agent for the control of specific outbreaks of infection.

2. Wear clean gloves when touching blood, body fluids, secretions, excretions, and contaminated items (for example, soiled gowns).

a. Clean gloves can be unsterile unless they are intended to prevent the entrance of microorganisms into the body.

b. Remove gloves before touching noncontaminated items and surfaces.

c. Wash hands immediately after removing gloves.

3. Wear a mask, eye protection, or a face shield if splashes or sprays of blood, body fluids, secretions, or excretions can be expected.

4. Wear a clean, nonsterile gown if client care is likely to result in splashes or sprays of blood, body fluids, secretions, or excretions. The gown is intended to protect clothing.

a. Remove a soiled gown carefully to avoid the transfer of microorganisms to others (for example, clients or other health care workers).

b. Wash hands after removing gown.

5. Handle client care equipment that is soiled with blood, body fluids, secretions, or excretions carefully to prevent the transfer of microorganisms to others and to the environment.

a. Make sure reusable equipment is cleaned and reprocessed correctly.

b. Dispose of single-use equipment correctly.

6. Handle, transport, and process linen that is soiled with blood, body fluids, secretions, or excretions in a manner to prevent contamination of clothing and the transfer of microorganisms to others and to the environment.

7. Prevent injuries from used equipment such as scalpels or needles, and place them in puncture-resistant containers.

Transmission-Based Precautions (Tier Two)

Airborne Precautions

Use the Tier One precautions as well as the following:

1. Place client in a private room that has negative air pressure, 6 to 12 air changes per hour and discharge of air to the outside or a filtration system for the room air.

2. If a private room is not available, place client with another client who is infected with the same microorganism.

3. Wear a respiratory device (N95 respirator) when entering the room of a client who is known or suspected of having primary tuberculosis.

4. Susceptible people should not enter the room of a client who has rubella (measles) or varicella (chickenpox). If they must enter they should wear a respirator.

5. Limit movement of client outside the room to essential purposes. Place a surgical mask on the client if possible.

Droplet Precautions

Use the Tier One precautions as well as the following:

1. Place client in private room.

2. If a private room is not available, place client with another client who is infected with the same microorganism.

3. Wear a mask if working within 3 feet of the client.

4. Transport client outside of the room only when necessary and place a surgical mask on the client if possible.

Contact Precautions

Use the Tier One precautions as well as the following:

1. Place client in private room.

2. If a private room is not available, place client with another client who is infected with the same microorganism.

3. Wear gloves as described in Standard Precautions.

   a. Change gloves after contact with infectious material.

   b. Remove gloves before leaving client's room.

   c. Wash hands immediately after removing gloves. Use an antimicrobial agent.

   d. After handwashing do not touch possibly contaminated surfaces or items in the room.

4. Wear a gown (see Standard Precautions) when entering a room if there is a possibility of contact with infected surfaces or items, or if the client is incontinent, has diarrhea, a colostomy, or wound drainage not contained by a dressing.

   a. Remove gown in the client's room.

   b. Make sure uniform does not contact possible contaminated surfaces.

5. Limit movement of client outside the room.

6. Dedicate the use of noncritical client care equipment to a single client or to clients with the same infecting microorganisms.

Source: Adapted from JS Garner and the Hospital Infection Control Practices Advisory Committee (HICPAC), Guidelines for isolation precautions in hospitals, *Infection Control Hospital Epidemiology,* 1996, 17:53–80 and NCID Home Page, February 18, 1997, and *American Journal of Infection Control,* 1996, 24:24–52.

B. COMPONENTS OF THE NURSING PROCESS

The nursing process is a systematic, rational method of planning and providing individualized nursing care. Its goal is to identify a client's health status and actual or potential health care problems, to establish plans to meet the identified needs, and to deliver specific nursing interventions to meet those needs. The nursing process is cyclical; that is, the components of the nursing process follow a logical sequence, but more than one component may be involved at any one time. There are five components of the nursing process:

1. *Assessing*—collecting, organizing, validating, and recording data about a client's health status to establish a database. Activities include obtaining a health history, performing a physical assessment, reviewing client records, reviewing literature, and consulting support people and health professionals.

2. *Diagnosing*—the process of analyzing and synthesizing data, which results in a diagnostic statement or nursing diagnosis. Activities include clustering data; comparing data against standards; generating tentative hypotheses; identifying gaps and inconsistencies; determining the

client's health strengths, risks, and problems; and formulating nursing diagnoses statements.

3. *Planning*—a series of steps in which the nurse and the client set priorities, goals, or desired outcomes and establish a written care plan designed to resolve or minimize the identified problems of the client and to coordinate the care provided by all health team members. Activities include setting priorities with the client, writing evaluation goals and outcome criteria with the client, selecting nursing strategies, consulting with other health care personnel, writing nursing orders and nursing care plans, and communicating the care plan to relevant health care providers.

4. *Implementing*—putting the nursing care plan into action to help the client attain goals. Activities include reassessing the client, updating the database, reviewing and revising the care plan, and performing or delegating planned nursing interventions.

5. *Evaluating*—measuring the degree to which goals/outcomes have been achieved and identifying factors that promote or impede goal achievement. Activities include collecting data about the client's response, comparing the client's response to evaluation criteria, relating nursing actions to client outcomes, making decisions about problem status, and modifying the care plan.

Refer to Chapters 17–21 of *Fundamentals of Nursing* for a thorough discussion of the components of the nursing process.

C. COMMUNICATION GUIDELINES

Communication is a vital part of nursing practice. Nurses who communicate effectively are better able to initiate change that promotes health, establish a trusting relationship with clients, families, and colleagues, and prevent legal problems associated with nursing practice. Effective communication is essential to establishing a positive nurse-client relationship. Refer to Chapter 25 of *Fundamentals of Nursing* for a thorough discussion of communication techniques.

Therapeutic communication techniques can help promote understanding between nurse and client. These techniques include the following:

- Being silent when appropriate
- Asking open-ended questions
- Using touch
- Restating or paraphrasing
- Seeking clarification
- Summarizing

In some situations, ordinary methods of communication are not sufficient, for example, when caring for a client who is angry, confused, or speaks a language foreign to you. Some cultural issues also require sensitivity and understanding.

The Angry Client

Anger can be the result of fear, frustration, or a feeling of losing control. Often clients direct their anger toward the nurse, simply because the nurse is there. Angry outbursts from clients may be due to worries about their job, family, or illness. Fatigue or physical discomfort can also provoke anger. It is important that you try to identify the cause of the anger and not to feed that anger; maintain your composure.

The following are guidelines for responding to the angry client:

- Listen to what the client is saying.

- Don't let the client's anger cause you to react and not listen.

- Use techniques such as reflection, clarification, and focusing to find out what the problem is. Only when you understand the problem can you formulate a plan for resolution.

- Once the problem is identified, find ways to resolve it. Remember, **don't make promises you can't keep.** A trusting relationship is key in diffusing angry outbursts.

- If you can't resolve the client's anger, or if there is any threat of violence, ask your instructor or the primary nurse for assistance.

- Be sure to document the conversation or incident, no matter how minor it may seem.

The Confused Client

Confusion in a client can be caused by medications, disease process, or the disruption of circadian rhythms. Whatever the cause, working with the confused client can be frustrating, so it is important to know your trigger points and what soothes them.

The following are guidelines for responding to the confused client:

- If this confusion is a new occurrence, review the client's medications and the potential side effects. Sudden onset of confusion is a sign that must be reported. Review your findings with your instructor.

- At every interaction with the client, orient the client to person, time, and place. Try to interact with the client as often as possible.

- Actively listen to the client, and clarify any points of confusion. Be attentive.

- Ask the family to orient the client as well. Be sensitive to the family's needs; they too can become frustrated.

- Reassure the client, but don't be condescending.

The Anxious Client

Fear of the unknown causes anxiety. All of us experience it at one time or another. As a nurse, it is important that you identify the causes or origin of a client's fear or anxiety.

The following are guidelines to use in responding to the anxious client:

- Talk to the client and actively listen. Answer all questions you can answer accurately. Use the skills of reflection, clarification, and focusing to get the client to talk about the true problem.

- Questions such as "Am I going to die?" or "Do I have AIDS or cancer?" are the most disconcerting. Ask clients what makes them believe that they are going to die or that they have AIDS or cancer. Your goal is to get them to verbalize their fears.

- If the client has questions about the diagnosis, find out what the client has already been told. Clarify any points you can. If the client has not been told anything, ask whether the client would like to speak to the physician. It is the physician's responsibility, not yours, to communicate the diagnosis.

- Be attentive to the client. Look in on the client as much as possible. This establishes trust and communicates a caring attitude.

- Above all, don't be condescending or dismiss the client's anxiety. Put yourself in the client's position.

Communicating Across Language Barriers

There are many types of language barriers. Foreign language, hearing deficits, expressive disorders (such as aphasia), and intubation are all barriers to effective communication and require some creativity, patience, and perseverance. It is crucial for the client to be able to communicate needs and for the nurse to be able to communicate understanding. Health care facilities usually have resources that can help you, such as translation services for the non-English-speaking client and for the hearing impaired. The speech therapy department can help you find ways to communicate with a client who has speech deficits.

The Non-English-Speaking Client

- Find out whether the health care facility has a translation service.

- Find out if any staff members speak the language.

- Contact local churches or ethnic organizations which may provide a translator.

- Don't yell at the client. Speaking more loudly may only make the patient think you are angry. If the client does not understand English, increasing the decibel level will not help.

- If a particular language is commonly spoken at the facility (for example, Spanish), purchase a phrase book and take the opportunity to add to your skills. You may also wish to develop a resource binder containing frequently used terms in many languages.

- If all else fails, act out what you are going to do. This does work.

- As a last resort, enlist the help of a family member or friend who may be able to translate. However, be considerate of these people; translating can be very stressful. Remember that they are the client's support system, not yours. Also, clients may be reluctant to share intimate health information with family members.

The Hearing-Impaired Client

- Stand in front of the hearing-impaired client and talk distinctly at a normal tone. Make sure the client can clearly see you. Many clients who are hard of hearing read lips.

- Keep paper and pencil at the bedside and write notes, especially when privacy is important.

- For the client who uses sign language, enlist the help of a translation service, if available.

- If no services are available to help you and writing is not possible, act out what you would like to do.

- Take the opportunity to learn sign language.

The Client with Aphasia

- Listen carefully. Encourage the client to take her time. Don't be afraid to ask the client to repeat herself.

- Use paper and pencil, or picture board, if appropriate.

- If the aphasia is a long-standing condition, ask a family member for assistance.

- Call the speech therapy department for any additional help, if needed.

The Intubated Client

- Use paper and pencil for communication or a letter board on which the client can spell out words.

- If yes or no answers are needed, have the client blink once for yes and twice for no.

Cultural Issues

In almost every area of the country, nurses come into contact with people from cultures different from their own. Although it is not within the scope of this book to describe the differences in all cultures you may encounter, there are some universal guidelines that can be of help.

Examine your own attitudes. What are your attitudes toward different cultures? What experiences have you had with different races and ethnic groups? What influences your acceptance or nonacceptance of a cultural group? Are your beliefs about a certain culture based on experience or on what you have heard or read? Refer to Chapter 13 of *Fundamentals of Nursing* for a thorough discussion of cultural issues.

The following are guidelines for responding to clients of different cultures:

- Always treat the client with respect.

- Different cultures may use different behaviors to denote respect or understanding. Do not assume you know the meaning of a specific behavior.

- Familiarize yourself with the customs and beliefs of cultural groups in your area.

- Try to incorporate cultural symbols and practices into the care plan of the client where feasible; these can bring comfort to a client.

- Remember that the color of a person's skin does not necessarily indicate the person's cultural background.

- Learn how the client views health, illness, grieving, and the health care system.

D. COMMON ABBREVIATIONS

Abbreviation	Term
abd	abdomen
ABO	the main blood group system
ac	before meals (ante cibum)
ADL	activities of daily living
ad lib	as desired (ad libitum)
adm	admitted or admission
AM	morning (ante meridiem)
amb	ambulatory
amt	amount
approx	approximately (about)
bid	twice daily (bis in die)
BM (bm)	bowel movement
BP	blood pressure
BR	bed rest
BRP	bathroom privileges
$\bar{c}$ (C)	with
C	Celsius (centigrade)
CBC	complete blood count
CBR	complete bed rest
Cl	client
c/o	complains of
DAT	diet as tolerated
dc (disc)	discontinue
DNR	do not resuscitate
drsg	dressing

Abbreviation	Term
Dx	diagnosis
ECG (EKG)	electrocardiogram
F	Fahrenheit
fld	fluid
GI	gastrointestinal
GP	general practitioner
gtt	drops (guttae)
h (hr)	hour (hora)
H_2O	water
hs	at bedtime (hora somni)
I & O	intake and output
IV	intravenous
Lab	laboratory
liq	liquid
LMP	last menstrual period
Lt (lt, L)	left
meds	medications
mL (ml)	milliliter
mod	moderate
neg	negative
nil (o)	none
no. (#)	number
NPO (NBM)	nothing by mouth (nil per os)
NS (N/S)	normal saline
O_2	oxygen
od	daily (omni die)
OD	right eye (oculus dexter); overdose
OOB	out of bed
os	mouth
OS	left eye (oculus sinister)
pc	after meals (post cibum)
PE (PX)	physical examination

→

D. Common Abbreviations *(continued)*

Abbreviation	Term
per	by or through
PM	afternoon (post meridiem)
po	by mouth (per os)
postop	postoperative(ly)
preop	preoperative(ly)
prep	preparation
prn	when necessary (pro re nata)
pt	patient
q	every (quaque)
qd	every day (quaque die)
qh (q1h)	every hour (quaque hora)
q2h, q3h, etc.	every 2 hours, 3 hours, etc.
qhs	every night at bedtime (quaque hora somni)
qid	four times a day (quater in die)
req	requisition
Rt (rt, R)	right
$\overline{s}$ (S)	without (sine)
spec	specimen
stat	at once, immediately (statim)
tid	three times a day (ter in die)
TL	team leader
TLC	tender loving care
TPR	temperature, pulse, respirations
Tr.	tincture
VO	verbal order
VS (vs)	vital signs
WNL	within normal limits
wt	weight

E. MEDICAL TERMINOLOGY: ROOT WORDS, PREFIXES, AND SUFFIXES

Word Element	Meaning
Root Words	
Circulatory System	
cardio	heart
angio, vaso	vessel
hem, hema, hemato	blood
vena, phlebo	vein
arteria	artery
lympho	lymph
thrombo	clot (of blood)
embolus	moving clot
Digestive System	
bucca	cheek
os, stomato	mouth
gingiva	gum
glossa	tongue
pharyngo	pharynx
esophago	esophagus
gastro	stomach
hepato	liver
cholecyst	gallbladder
pancreas	pancreas
entero	intestines
duodeno	duodenum

→

E. Medical Terminology *(continued)*

Word Element	Meaning
Root Words	
jejuno	jejunum
ileo	ileum
caeco	cecum
appendeco	appendix
colo	colon
recto	rectum
ano, procto	anus
Skeletal System	
skeleto	skeleton
Respiratory System	
naso, rhino	nose
tonsillo	tonsil
laryngo	larynx
tracheo	trachea
bronchus, broncho	bronchus (pl. bronchi)
pulmo, pneuma, pneum	lung (sac with air)
Nervous System	
neuro	nerve
cerebrum	brain
oculo, ophthalmo	eye
oto	ear
psych, psycho	mind
Urinary System	
urethro	urethra
cysto	bladder
uretero	ureter
reni, reno, nephro	kidney
pyleo	pelvis of kidney
uro	urine

Word Element	Meaning
Female Reproductive System	
vulvo	vulva
perineo	perineum
labio	labium (pl. labia)
vagino, colpo	vagina
cervico	cervix
utero	womb; uterus
tubo, salpingo	fallopian tube
ovario, oophoro	ovary
Male Reproductive System	
orchido	testes
Regions of the Body	
crani, cephalo	head
cervico, tracheo	neck
thoraco	chest
abdomino	abdomen
dorsum	back
Tissues	
cutis, dermato	skin
lipo	fat
musculo, myo	muscle
osteo	bone
myelo	marrow
chrondro	cartilage
Miscellaneous	
cyto	cell
genetic	formation, origin
gram	tracing or mark
graph	writing, description
kinesis	motion
meter	measure
oligo	small, few

→

E. Medical Terminology *(continued)*

Word Element	Meaning
Root Words	
phobia	fear
photo	light
pyo	pus
scope	instrument for visual examination
roentgen	x-ray
lapar	flank; through the abdominal wall

Prefixes	
a, an, ar	without or not
ab	away from
acro	extremities
ad	toward, to
adeno	glandular
aero	air
ambi	around, on both sides
amyl	starch
ante	before, forward
anti	against, counteracting
bi	double
bili	bile
bio	life
bis	two
brachio	arm
brady	slow
broncho	bronchus (pl. bronchi)
cardio	heart
cervico	neck
chole	gall or bile
cholecysto	gall bladder
circum	around
co	together

Word Element	Meaning
contra	against, opposite
costo	ribs
cyto	cell
cysto	bladder
demi	half
derma	skin
dis	from
dorso	back
dys	abnormal, difficult
electro	electric
en	into, in, within
encephal	brain
entero	intestine
equi	equal
eryth	red
ex	out, out of, away from
extra	outside of, in addition to
ferro	iron
fibro	fiber
fore	before, in front of
gastro	stomach
glosso	tongue
glyco	sugar
hemi	half
hemo	blood
hepa, hepato	liver
histo	tissue
homo	same
hydro	water
hygro	moisture
hyper	too much, high
hypo	under, decreased
hyster	uterus
ileo	ileum

→

E. Medical Terminology (continued)

Word Element	Meaning
Prefixes	
in	in, within, into
inter	between
intra	within
intro	in, within, into
juxta	near, close to
laryngo	larynx
latero	side
lapar	abdomen
leuk	white
macro	large, big
mal	bad, poor
mast	breast
medio	middle
mega, megalo	large, great
meno	menses
mono	single
multi	many
myelo	bone marrow, spinal cord
myo	muscle
neo	new
nephro	kidney
neuro	nerve
nitro	nitrogen
noct	night
non	not
ob	against, in front of
oculo	eye
odonto	tooth
ophthalmo	eye
ortho	straight, normal
os	mouth, bone

Word Element	Meaning
osteo	bone
oto	ear
pan	all
para	beside, accessory to
path	disease
ped	child, foot
per	by, through
peri	around
pharyngo	pharynx
phlebo	vein
photo	light
phren	diaphragm, mind
pneumo	air, lungs
pod	foot
poly	many, much
post	after
pre	before
proct	rectum
pseudo	false
psych	mind
pyel	pelvis of the kidney
pyo	pus
pyro	fever, heat
quadri	four
radio	radiation
re	back, again
reno	kidney
retro	backward
rhin	nose
sacro	sacrum
salpingo	fallopian tube
sarco	flesh
sclero	hard, hardening
semi	half

→

E. Medical Terminology *(continued)*

Word Element	Meaning
Prefixes	
sex	six
skeleto	skeleton
steno	narrowing, constriction
sub	under
super	above, excess
supra	above
syn	together
tachy	fast
thyro	thyroid, gland
trache	trachea
trans	across, over
tri	three
ultra	beyond
un	not, back, reversal
uni	one
uretero	ureter
urethro	urethra
uro	urine, urinary organs
vaso	vessel
Suffixes	
able	able to
algia	pain
cele	tumor, swelling
centesis	surgical pucture to remove fluid
cide	killing, destructive
cule	little
cyte	cell
ectasia	dilating, stretching
ectomy	excision, surgical removal of
emia	blood
esis	action

Word Element	Meaning
form	shaped like
genesis, genetic	formation, origin
gram	tracing, mark
graph	writing
ism	condition
itis	inflammation
ize	to treat
lith	stone, calculus
lithiasis	presence of stones
lysis	disintegration
megaly	enlargement
meter	instrument that measures
oid	likeness, resemblance
oma	tumor
opathy	disease of
orrhaphy	surgical repair
osis	disease, condition of
ostomy	to form an opening or outlet
otomy	to incise
pexy	fixation
phage	ingesting
phobia	fear
plasty	plastic surgery
plegia	paralysis
rhage	to burst forth
rhea	excessive discharge
rhexis	rupture
scope	lighted instrument for visual examination
scopy	to examine visually
stomy	to form an opening
tomy	incision into
uria	urine

F. WEIGHT AND VOLUME CONVERSIONS AND EQUIVALENTS

Prefix	Abbreviations	Numerical	Value
Basic Metric Units			
kilo	k	1000	(one thousand)
hecto	h	100	(one hundred)
deka	dk	10	(ten)
deci	d	0.1	(one-tenth)
centi	c	0.01	(one-hundredth)
milli	m	0.001	(one-thousandth)
micro	mc,μ	0.000001	(one-millionth)

Metric Weight Equivalents	
1 kg (kilogram)	= 1000 g (grams)
1 g (gram)	= 1000 mg (milligrams)
1 mg (milligram)	= 1000 mcg,μg (micrograms)

Approximate Weight Equivalents:
Metric and Apothecaries' Systems

Metric	Apothecaries'
0.1 mg	1/600 grain (gr)
0.6 mg	1/100 grain
1 mg	1/60 grain
4 mg	1/15 grain
6 mg	1/10 grain
10 mg	1/6 grain

Metric	Apothecaries'
15 mg	1/4 grain
30 mg	1/2 grain
60 mg	1 grain
500 mg (0.5 g)	7 1/2 grains
600 mg (0.6 g)	10 grains
1 gram (1000 mg)	15 grains
2 g	30 grains
4 g	60 grains (1 dram)
7.5 g	120 grains (2 drams)
30 g	1 ounce (8 drams)
1000 g	2.2 pounds (1 kilogram)

Approximate Volume Equivalents:
Metric, Apothecaries', and
Household Systems

Metric	Apothecaries'	Household
0.06 mL	1 minim (m)	1 drop (gt)
0.3 mL	5 minims	5 drops (gtt)
0.6 mL	10 minims	10 drops (gtt)
1 mL (1 cubic cm.)	15 minims	15 drops (gtt)
2 mL	30 minims	30 drops (gtt)
3 mL	45 minims	45 drops (gtt)
4 mL	60 minims (1 fluid dram [ʒ])	60 drops (1 teaspoon [tsp])
8 mL	2 fluid drams	2 teaspoons
15 mL	4 fluid drams	4 teaspoons (1 tablespoon [Tbsp])
30 mL	8 fluid drams (1 fluid ounce [ʒ])	2 tablespoons
60 mL	2 fluid ounces	
90 mL	3 fluid ounces	
200 mL	6 fluid ounces	1 teacup
250 mL	8 fluid ounces	1 large glass

→

F. Weight and Volume
Conversions and Equivalents *(continued)*

Approximate Volume Equivalents:
Metric, Apothecaries', and
Household Systems

Metric	Apothecaries'	Household
500 mL	16 fluid ounces (1 pint [pt])	1 pint
1000 mL (1 liter)	2 pints (1 quart [qt])	1 quart
4000 mL 1 gallon (gal)	4 quarts	

G. LABORATORY VALUES

The ranges for normal values may vary from laboratory to laboratory; therefore, always check with each agency for its own normal range and for the particular testing method, and, if indicated, for the population for which the set of values is described. All values should be interpreted within the context of the client's health status. Refer to Chapter 48 of *Fundamentals of Nursing* for a thorough discussion of fluids, electrolytes, and acid-base balance.

Table A: Serum, Plasma, and Whole Blood Chemistries

Test	NORMAL VALUES Conventional Units	SI Units	POSSIBLE ETIOLOGIES Higher	Lower
Amylase	60 to 160 U/L (method dependent)	30 to 170 U/L	Cholecystitis, diabetic ketoacidosis, ectopic pregnancy, pancreatic cancer, pancreatitis, salivary gland disease (eg, mumps)	Burns (severe), cirrhosis of liver, hepatitis, extensive destruction of pancreas, thyrotoxicosis (severe), toxemia of pregnancy

→

Table A: Serum, Plasma, and Whole Blood Chemistries (*continued*)

Test	NORMAL VALUES Conventional Units	SI Units	POSSIBLE ETIOLOGIES Higher	Lower
Bilirubin				
Total	0.1 to 1.2 mg/dL	1.7 to 20.5 μmol/L	Anemia (hemolytic or pernicious), biliary obstruction, drug reactions (eg, to chlorpromazine), fasting (prolonged), impaired hepatic function, infectious mononucleosis, multiple transfusions, transfusion reactions	Iron-deficiency anemia
Indirect	0.1 to 1.0 mg/dL	1.7 to 17.1 μmol/L		—
Direct	0.1 to 0.3 mg/dL	1.7 to 5.1 μmol/L		—

Blood gases*	Conventional units	Conventional units	Alkalosis (metabolic and respiratory)	Acidosis (metabolic and respiratory)
Venous pH	7.35 to 7.45 7.31 to 7.45			
Arterial Pco$_2$	35 to 45 mm Hg	4.67 to 6.00 kPa	Compensated metabolic alkalosis or respiratory acidosis	Compensated metabolic acidosis or respiratory alkalosis
Arterial Po$_2$	> 80 mm Hg	10.0 to 13.33 kPa	Administration of high concentration of oxygen	Chronic lung disease, anemia
Arterial Hco$_3$	22 to 26 mEqL	20 to 30 mmol/L	Metabolic alkalosis	Metabolic acidosis
Bass excess (BE)	−2 to +2 mEqL	—	Metabolic alkalosis	Metabolic acidosis
Calcium	4.3 to 5.3 mEq/L Total:8.8 to 10.0 mg/dL	2.3 to 2.8 mmol/L	Acromegaly, cancer metastasis to bone, acute osteoporosis, hyperparathyroidism, multiple myeloma, vitamin D intoxication	Acute pancreatitis, hepatic disease, hypoparathyroidism, malabsorption syndrome, renal failure, vitamin D deficiency

→

Table A: Serum, Plasma, and Whole Blood Chemistries (*continued*)

Test	NORMAL VALUES Conventional Units	SI Units	POSSIBLE ETIOLOGIES Higher	Lower
Chloride	95 to 105 mEq/L	95 to 105 mmol/L	Cardiac decompensation, dehydration, hypernatremia, metabolic acidosis, respiratory alkalosis, steroid therapy, uremia	Addison's disease, burns (severe), diarrhea, diuretic use, metabolic alkalosis, respiratory acidosis, vomiting, gastric suctioning
Cholesterol Desirable level Moderate risk High risk	<200 mg/dL 200 to 240 mg/dL >240 mg/dL	Conventional units Conventional units	Atherosclerosis, biliary obstruction, diabetes (uncontrolled), hypertension, hypothyroidism, idiopathic hypercholesterolemia, myocardial infarction, pregnancy, renal disease	Anemia, hepatic disease (extensive), hyperthyroidism, malnutrition, sepsis, steroid therapy, starvation, malabsorption

Test	Conventional units	SI units	Increased	Decreased
Creatine phosphokinase (CPK) or creatine kinase (CK)			Muscular dystrophy, musculoskeletal injury or disease, myocardial infarction, myocarditis (severe), numerous intramuscular injections, brain damage, pulmonary infarction, chronic alcoholism, electric shock	
Male	55 to 170 U/L	Conventional units		—
Female	30 to 135 U/L (method dependent)	Conventional units		—
Creatinine	0.5 to 1.5 mg/dL	45 to 133 μmol/L	Cancer, congestive heart failure, Hodgkin's disease, shock, leukemia, renal disease	Myasthenia gravis, muscular dystrophy, toxemia of pregnancy

→

Table A: Serum, Plasma, and Whole Blood Chemistries (*continued*)

Test	NORMAL VALUES Conventional Units	SI Units	POSSIBLE ETIOLOGIES Higher	Lower
Glucose, fasting Serum Whole blood	70 to 110 mg/dL 60 to 105 mg/dL	3.9 to 6.11 mmol/L 3.3 to 5.81 mmol/L	Cerebral lesions, Cushing's syndrome, diabetes mellitus, hyperthyroidism, pancreatic insufficiency, stress (acute)	Addison's disease, hepatic disease, hypothyroidism, insulin overdose, pancreatic tumor, pituitary hypofunction, postgastrectomy dumping syndrome
Lactic dehydrogenase (LDH)	70 to 250 U/L at 30C (varies considerably with method used)	Conventional units	Cerebrovascular accident, collagen diseases, hemolytic disorders, liver disease, myocardial infarction, pernicious anemia, pulmonary embolus, skeletal muscle damage	—

Magnesium	1.3 to 2.1 mEq/L	Conventional units	Addison's disease, dehydration, diabetic ketoacidosis, excessive use of antacids, hypothyroidism, leukemia, renal disorders	Chronic alcoholism, chronic diarrhea, chronic renal disease, gastric suctioning, hypoparathyroidism, hyperthyroidism, severe malabsorption, toxemia of pregnancy
Osmolality	280 to 300 mOsm/kg	Conventional units	Chronic renal disease, diabetes insipidus, diabetes mellitus, fluid volume deficit	Acute renal disease, Addison's disease, diuretic therapy, fluid volume excess, syndrome of inappropriate antidiuretic hormone secretion (SIADH)

→

Table A: Serum, Plasma, and Whole Blood Chemistries (*continued*)

Test	NORMAL VALUES Conventional Units	SI Units	POSSIBLE ETIOLOGIES Higher	Lower
Oxygen saturation (arterial)	95% to 98%	0.95 to 0.98 saturated	Polycythemia	Anemia, cardiac decompensation, respiratory disorders
Phosphorus, inorganic Male Female	2.8 to 4.5 mg/dL 1.7 to 2.6 mg/dL 2.5 to 4.5 mg/dL	0.90 to 1.45 mmol/L	Healing fractures, hypocalcemia, hypoparathyroidism, renal disease, skeletal disease, vitamin D intoxication	Chronic alcoholism, continuous dextrose infusions, diabetes mellitus, hypercalcemia, hyperparathyroidism, vitamin D deficiency, prolonged gastric suctioning, vomiting

Potassium	3.5 to 5.0 mEq/L	3.5 to 5.0 mmol/L	Acidosis, Addison's disease, diabetic ketosis, hypoaldosteronism, massive tissue destruction, renal failure, use of potassium-sparing diuretics	Alkalosis, Cushing's syndrome, diarrhea (severe), diuretic therapy, gastrointestinal fistula, pyloric obstruction, starvation, vomiting
Proteins		Conventional units		
Total	6.0 to 8.0 g/dL	60 to 80 g/L		
Albumin	3.2 to 5.0 g/dL	35 to 50 g/L		
Globulin	2.0 to 3.5 g/dL	20 to 35 g/L	Burns, cirrhosis (globulin fraction), dehydration, hemoconcentration	Ascites, congenital agammaglobulinemia, hepatic disease, lupus erythematosus, malabsorption
Albimin/globulin ratio	1.5:1 to 2.5:1		Multiple myeloma (globulin fraction), shock, vomiting	Burns (severe), malnutrition, nephrotic syndrome, proteinuria, renal disease

→

Table A: Serum, Plasma, and Whole Blood Chemistries (continued)

Test	NORMAL VALUES Conventional Units	SI Units	POSSIBLE ETIOLOGIES Higher	Lower
Sodium	136 to 148 mEq/L	136 to 148 mmol/L	Cushing's syndrome, dehydration, diabetes insipidus, impaired renal function, primary aldosteronism, steroid therapy, free water loss (eg, sweat), use of osmotic diuretics	Addison's disease, bowel obstruction, diabetic ketoacidosis, diuretic therapy, excessive gastrointestinal tract loss, excessive perspiration, IV therapy, water intoxication
Urea nitrogen (BUN)	7 to 18 mg/dL	2.5 to 6.3 mmol/L	Diabetes mellitus, increase in protein catabolism (fever, stress) or excessive protein intake, renal disease, urinary tract infection	Malnutrition, overhydration, severe liver damage

Uric acid			
Male	3.5 to 8.0 mg/dL	Acute infectious mononucleosis, alcoholism, chemotherapy, eclampsia, gout, gross tissue destruction, high-protein weight reduction diet, leukemia, metastatic cancer, renal failure	Administration of uricosuric drugs
Female	2.8 to 6.8 mg/dL		

*Because arterial blood gases are influenced by altitude, the value for PO_2 decreases as altitude increases. The lower value is normal for an altitude of 1 mile.

†Values depend on reagent used.

††Components of complete blood count (CBC).

Table B: Hematologic Values

Test	NORMAL VALUES Conventional Units	SI Units	POSSIBLE ETIOLOGIES Higher	Lower
Partial thromboplastin time (PTT)	60 to 70 sec (hemophilia is a factor VIII deficiency)	—	Factor deficiencies, cirrhosis, vitamin K deficiency, disseminated intravascular coagulation (DIC)	Extensive cancer
Activated partial; thromboplastin time (APTT)	20 to 35 sec[†] 1.5 to 2.5 times control when receiving anticoagulants	Conventional units	Deficiency of clotting factors I, II, V, VIII, IX, and X, XI, XII; disseminated intravascular coagulation (DIC); heparin therapy; hepatic disease; leukemia; von Willebrand's disease	Early-state DIC

Test		Conventional units	Increased	Decreased
Prothombin time (Protime, PT)	10 to 14 sec†		Anticoagulant therapy; biliary obstruction; deficiency of factors I, II, V, VII, and X; DIC; hepatic liver disease; salicylate toxicity; vitamin K deficiency in diet	Thrombophlebitis, pulmonary embolism, myocardial infarction
Erythrocyte (red blood cell) count (altitude dependent)			Congenital heart disease, cor pulmonale, dehydration, diarrhea (severe), high altitudes, polycythemia vera	Anemia, Addison's disease, leukemia, lupus erythematosus, multiple myeloma, organ failure, pregnancy
Male	4.2 to $6.0 \times 10^6/\mu l$	4.2 to $6.0 \times 10^{12}/\mu l$		
Female	3.6 to $5.0 \times 10^6/\mu l$	3.6 to $5.0 \times 10^{12}/\mu l$		

→

Table B: Hematologic Values (continued)

Test	NORMAL VALUES Conventional Units	SI Units	POSSIBLE ETIOLOGIES Higher	Lower
Erythrocyte sedimentation rate (ESR)			Moderate increase: acute hepatitis, myocardial infarction, rheumatoid arthritis; marked increase: acute and severe bacterial infections, acute myocardial infarction, collagen diseases, malignancies, pelvic inflammatory disease, pneumonia, toxemia	Angina pectoris, congestive heart failure, degenerative arthritis, hepatic disease (severe), infectious mononucleosis, malaria, polycythemia vera, sickle-cell anemia
Male	<15mm/h	Conventional units		
Female	<20 mm/h (method dependent)	Conventional units		
Hematocrit (altitude dependent)[††]			Dehydration, eclampsia, high altitudes, polycythemia, shock, surgery/trauma	Anemia, bone marrow dysfunction, cirrhosis, hemorrhage, hemolytic reactions, leukemia, malnutrition, overhydration, pregnancy
Male	40% to 54%	0.40 to 0.54		
Female	38% to 47%	0.38 to 0.47		

Hemoglobin (altitude dependent)[++]			
Male	13.5 to 18.0 g/dL	8.7 to 11.31 mmol/L	Chronic obstructive pulmonary disease (COPD), congestive heart failure (CHF), hemoconcentration, high altitudes, polycythemia	Hemolytic reactions, hemorrhage, iron deficiency anemia, leukemia, renal disease, sickle-cell disease, systemic lupus erythematosus
Female	12.0 to 16.0 g/dL	7.4 to 9.9 mmol/L		
Platelet count (thrombocytes)[++]	150,000 to 400,000/µl	150 to 400 × 10^9/L	Acute infections, chronic pancreatitis, chronic rheumatoid arthritis, cirrhosis, collagen disorders, leukemia, polycythemia, postsplenectomy	Cancer chemotherapy, disseminated intravascular coagulation (DIC), hemolytic anemia, hepatic liver disease, leukemia (acute), systemic lupus erythematosus, thrombocytopenic purpura

→

Table B: Hematologic Values (continued)

Test	NORMAL VALUES Conventional Units	SI Units	POSSIBLE ETIOLOGIES Higher	Lower
Reticulocyte count	0.5% to 1.5% of RBC	25,000 to 75,000 μL	Hemolytic anemia, polycythemia vera, pregnancy, sickle-cell anemia	Hypoproliferative anemia, macrocytic anemia, microcytic anemia
White blood cell count (total) Monocytes Basophils	4 to 11,000/μL	4.0 to 11.0 × 10⁹/L	Inflammatory and infectious processes, leukemia, tissue necrosis	Aplastic anemia, autoimmune disease, bone marrow failure, chemotherapy, drug toxicity (eg, chloramphenicol), overwhelming infection, radiation therapy

WBC differential			
Total neutrophils	50% to 70%	Bacterial infections, collagen diseases, Cushing's syndrome, eclampsia, gout, Hodgkin's disease, inflammatory disease, myelo-ketoacidosis, myelocytic leukemia, stress	Addison's disease, aplastic anemia, autoimmune disease, overwhelming infection (esp. in elderly), viral infection
Segments	50% to 65%		
Band neutrophils	0% to 5%	Acute infections	—
Lymphocytes	25% to 35%	Chronic infections, hepatitis, lymphocytic leukemia, mononucleosis, multiple myeloma, viral infections	Adrenocortico steriod therapy, Hodgkin's disease, immunodeficiency, leukemia, lupus erythematosus, sepsis, whole body iradiation

→

Table B: Hematologic Values (continued)

Test	NORMAL VALUES Conventional Units	SI Units	POSSIBLE ETIOLOGIES Higher	Lower
Monocytes	4% to 6%	0.02 to 0.08	Chronic inflammatory disorders, malaria, monocytic leukemia, tuberculosis, viral infections	Prednisone therapy
Eosinophils	1% to 3%	0.01 to 0.04 0.005 to 0.02	Allergic reactions, autoimmune disease, eczema, eosinophilic and chronic granulo-cytic leukemia, parasitic disorders	Steroid therapy Anaphylactic reaction, hypothyroidism, stress reactions
Basophils	0.4% to 1.0%	0.005 to 0.02	Acute severe infections, myolo-leukemia, myolo-proliferative diseases	

†Values depend on reagent used.
††Components of complete blood count (CBC).

Table C: Urine Chemistry

Test	Specimen	NORMAL VALUES Conventional Units	SI Units	POSSIBLE ETIOLOGIES Higher	Lower
Bilirubin	Random	Negative	Conventional units	Cirrhosis, gallstone, hepatic obstruction, hepatitis	—
Calcium	24h	100 to 250 mg/day	2.5 to 6.3 mmol/day	Bone tumor, hyperparathyroidism, milk-alkali syndrome	Calcium and vitamin D malabsorption, hypoparathyroidism, renal disease
Creatinine Male	24h	0.8 to 2.0 g/day	7.1 to 17.7 mmol/day	Anemia, leukemia, muscular atrophy, salmonella infection, tissue catabolism	Congestive heart failure (CHF), nephrotoxic drugs, renal disease, shock
Female		0.6 to 1.8 g/day	5.3 to 15.9 mmol/day		

→

Table C: Urine Chemistry (continued)

Test	Specimen	NORMAL VALUES Conventional Units	SI Units	POSSIBLE ETIOLOGIES Higher	Lower
Creatinine clearance	24h				Amyotrophic lateral sclerosis (ALS), CHF, drug toxicity, hyperthyroidism, multiple sclerosis, renal disease, shock
Male		70 to 150 mL/min	1.42 to 2.25 mL/sec	Exercise, hypothyroidism, renovascular hypertension	
Female		85 to 132 mL/min	1.42 to 2.25 mL/sec		
Glucose	Random	Negative	Conventional units	Cushing's syndrome, diabetes mellitus, infection, low renal threshold for glucose resorption, physiologic stress, pituitary disorders, pregnancy	—

		Conventional units	
Hemoglobin Random	Negative	Negative	Burns (extensive), glomerulonephritis, hemolytic anemias, hemolytic transfusion reaction, lupus erythematosus, malignant hypertension, urinary tract infections
Ketone bodies Random dipstick	Negative	Negative	Diabetes (uncontrolled), fasting, high-protein diet, starvation, vomiting (prolonged)

→

Table C: Urine Chemistry (continued)

Test	Specimen	NORMAL VALUES Conventional Units	SI Units	POSSIBLE ETIOLOGIES Higher	Lower
pH	Random	4.0 to 8.0	Conventional units	Alkalosis, chronic renal failure, diuretic use, gastric suction, salicylate intoxication, urinary tract infection, vegetable diet, vomiting	Acidosis, dehydration, diabetes mellitus, emphysema, starvation
Protein (dipstick)	Random	Negative	Conventional units	CHF, glomerulosclerosis, lupus erythematosus, multiple myeloma, nephrotic syndrome, physiologic stress, preeclampsia	—

		Conventional units			
Specific gravity	Random	1.010 to 1.025		Albuminuria, dehydration, diarrhea, glycosuria, presence of contrast medium, vomiting	Diabetes insipidus, overhydration, renal disease
Uric acid	24h	250 to 750 mg/day	1.5 to 4.5 mmol/day	Chronic alcohol ingestion, gout, hepatic disease, leukemia, toxemia of pregnancy, ulcerative colitis	Chronic glomerulonephritis, eclampsia, lead toxicity, nephritis, urinary obstruction

References

Kee, J. 1999. *Laboratory and Diagnostic Tests with Nursing Implications.* 5th ed. Norwalk, CT: Appleton & Lange.

LeMone, P and Burke, K. 2000. *Medical-Surgical Nursing.* 2nd ed. Menlo Park, CA: Addison-Wesley Nursing.

Pagana, K and Pagana, T. 1998. *Diagnostic Testing and Nursing Implications: A Case Study Approach.* 5th ed. St Louis: Mosby.

Seidel, H, Ball, J, Dains, J, and Benedict, G. 1990. *Mosby's Guide to Physical Examination.* 2d ed. St Louis: Mosby.

H. COMMON DIAGNOSTIC STUDIES

Test	Purpose
Blood	
Complete blood count (CBC)	To determine hemoglobin (Hgb), hematocrit (Hct), and erythrocyte, or red blood cell (RBC) count, and assess the blood's ability to carry oxygen. To determine the leukocyte, or white blood cell (WBC) count, which signals infection when elevated.
Serum electrolytes (Na^+, K^+, Mg^{2+}, Ca^{2+}, H^+)	To determine electrolyte and acid-base imbalances.
Arterial blood gas (ABG) analysis	To determine the adequacy of aleveolar gas exchange and evaluate the ability of the lungs and kidneys to maintain the acid-base balance of the body fluids. ABGs include pH, Pco2, bicarbonate, Po2 and O2 saturation and base excess.
Fasting blood sugar (FBS) test	To detect presence of glucose in the blood, which may indicate metabolic disorders (eg, diabetes mellitus).

→

H. Common Diagnostic Studies *(continued)*

Test	Purpose
Blood	
Glucose tolerance test (GTT)	To determine ability to tolerate a standard glucose load (insulin response) without spillage over into the urine.
Blood urea nitrogen (BUN) or creatinine	To assess urinary excretion.
Sputum	
Sputum culture and sensitivity test	To determine the presence of pathogenic bacteria and bacterial sensitivity to various antibiotics.
Acid-fast bacilli (AFB) test	To determine the presence of acid-fast bacilli indicating, for example, active tuberculosis.
Cytologic tests	To determine the presence of abnormal or malignant cells.
Urine	
Urinalysis (UA)	To detect urinary tract infections and glucose in the urine.
Urine culture and sensitivity test	To determine the presence of pathogenic bacteria and bacterial sensitivity to various antibiotics.
Stool	
Guaiac test	To determine the presence of occult blood and bleeding in the gastrointestinal tract.

Test	Purpose
Stool	
Ova and parasite tests	To determine the presence of a parasitic infection of the intestine.
Radiologic	
Chest roentgenogram (CXR)	To identify lung disease and heart size and location.
Upper gastrointestinal (UGI) test	To identify lesions in the esophagus, stomach, and duodenum after barium, a contrast medium, is swallowed.
Lower gastrointestinal (LGI) test	To identify lesions of the large bowel following a barium enema.
Scan of the head, chest, bone, or entire body	A noninvasive x-ray procedure that distinguishes minor differences in the radiodensity of soft tissues (eg, a tumor in liver tissue).
Other	
Electrocardiogram (ECG or EKG)	To determine the presence of cardiac disease.
Exercise stress test	To determine the client's ability to obtain and maintain maximum heart rate of 85% for predicted age and sex with no cardiac symptoms or EKG (ECG) change.
Tuberculin (TB) skin test	To detect tuberculosis infection; however, does not indicate whether the infection is active or dormant.

I. NURSING INTERVENTIONS FOR ENDOSCOPIC EXAMINATIONS

Examination	Preprocedure	NURSING INTERVENTION During Procedure	NURSING INTERVENTION Postprocedure
Laryngoscopy or bronchoscopy	Explain the procedure, and clarify the client's concerns. Explain that a local spray or gargle will be given or that medications will be injected through a needle in the vein; that the client will rest the teeth against a small plastic mouthpiece; and that the procedure is painless but some pressure may be felt. Explain that the test will take about 30 to 60 minutes. Assess vital signs, sputum, and character of respirations for baseline data. Remove dentures, necklaces, earrings, hairpins, and combs.	Assist the physician as required, for example, to hold the headpiece or to move the client's head. Monitor the client's pulse and respirations. Support the client using touch and verbal communication.	1. Monitor vital signs q30 minutes or as needed during the recovery period, and compare results to baseline data. 2. Withhold fluids until the gag reflex is restored and the client is conscious. 3. Position the client as ordered or indicated. Place the unconscious client in the lateral position so that secretions are not aspirated. 4. Inspect the client's sputum for blood caused by tissue damage.

5. Observe the client for signs of dyspnea, stridor, and shortness of breath, which may result from laryngeal edema or laryngospasm.
6. Provide ice chips and warm saline gargles or throat lozenges, and administer ordered analgesics as required for throat discomfort.
7. Advise the client to contact the physician should difficulty with breathing, blood in sputum, fever, or pain occur.

	Ensure good oral hygiene. Ensure that client is NPO for 6 to 8 hours beforehand. Confirm that the client is not allergic to any medications that will be given. Administer analgesic, sedative, antianxiety agent, and medication to dry secretions, if ordered.	As above for bronchoscopy. Administer oral simethicone (Mylicon) before test if ordered; it decreases air bubbles in the stomach.
Esophagoscopy, gastroscopy, and duodenoscopy	As above for bronchoscopy, with the exception of assessing sputum.	1. Follow steps 1 to 3 and 6, as for bronchoscopy.
		2. Inspect vomitus for blood, and test it for occult blood if agency practice indicates.

→

I. Nursing Interventions for Endoscopic Examinations (continued)

Examination	Preprocedure	NURSING INTERVENTION During Procedure	NURSING INTERVENTION Postprocedure
Esophagoscopy, gastroscopy, and duodenoscopy (continued)	Explain that the client may feel pressure in the stomach as the tube is moved about and feel fullness or bloating, like that after eating a large meal.	If atropine is given intravenously to reduce gastrointestinal spasm, carefully monitor the client's pulse rate. Atropine increases the heart rate.	3. Advise the client to contact the physician if client experiences persistent difficulty swallowing, pain, fever, blood in vomitus, or black stools.
Cystoscopy	Assess vital signs, frequency of urination, dysuria, and amount and consistency of urine for baseline data. Administer enema, if ordered. A clear bowel is necessary if x-ray studies are planned. If a general anesthetic is being given, ensure that client is NPO for 6 to 8 hours beforehand.	Support the client emotionally. Monitor vital signs. Label appropriately any specimens taken. Assist the physician as requested.	1. Monitor vital signs, urination, and urine, and compare with baseline data. 2. Position the unconscious client appropriately (as for bronchoscopy). 3. Inspect the client's urine for blood; report bright red bleeding. 4. Report inability to urinate by 8 hours.

	For the client having a local anesthetic, provide appropriate fluid intake, if ordered, to ensure an adequate flow of urine for the collection of specimens. Administer sedative and medication to dry secretions, if ordered.		5. Encourage increased fluid intake to decrease irritation of urinary tissue. 6. If dyes were used in the procedure, warn the client that the urine may be an unusual color. 7. Administer analgesics, as ordered. 8. Advise the client to report persistent difficulty passing urine, bright blood in urine, pain, or fever.
Anoscopy, proctoscopy, sigmoidoscopy, and colonoscopy	Assess vital signs and consistency of feces for baseline data. Ensure appropriate preexamination diet and fluid intake. Administer enemas until returns are clear, or suppository as ordered, the morning of the examination.	Support the client physically in the genupectoral position, as needed. Monitor pulse and respiratory rates. Label appropriately any specimens taken.	1. Monitor vital signs and compare with baseline data. 2. Inspect the next few bowel movements for blood. 3. Allow the client to rest. This procedure may be physically and emotionally tiring. 4. Provide fluids and food.

→

I. Nursing Interventions for Endoscopic Examinations (*continued*)

Examination	Preprocedure	NURSING INTERVENTION During Procedure	NURSING INTERVENTION Postprocedure
Anoscopy, proctoscopy, sigmoidoscopy, and colonoscopy (continued)	Ensure that the client voids before the examination. The pressure during the procedure may injure a full bladder. Administer sedative beforehand, if ordered. Just before the endoscope is inserted, explain that the client may experience (a) sensation of having to move bowels (due to the pressure of the instrument) and (b) abdominal cramping when distending bowel with air.	Support the client emotionally. Acknowledge feelings the client experiences (eg, cramps) and assure the client that they are not unusual.	

J. STUDIES OF THE GASTROINTESTINAL TRACT

Name	Description	NURSING INTERVENTION Preprocedure	NURSING INTERVENTION Postprocedure
Barium swallow	The client swallows barium, and the pharynx and esophagus are outlined on x-ray film.	Procedure lasts 30 minutes. Client is given a chalky substance (liquid barium) to drink.	Encourage fluids and activity to prevent constipation. Observe stool for whitish color, indicating client has passed barium in stool. Notify physician if barium not passed in 2 to 3 days (a laxative may be required.)
Upper gastrointestinal (UGI) series	The client swallows barium, and x-ray films are taken of its course through the esophagus, stomach, and duodenum.	Client must fast 4 to 6 hours before the examination. The client is given a chalky substance (liquid barium) to drink. Procedure lasts from 30 minutes to 1 hour. Client may experience a feeling of fullness. Client may need to assume several positions on the x-ray table.	Encourage fluids and activity to prevent constipation. Observe stool for whitish color, indicating client has passed barium in stool. Client may require a laxative or enema if client is constipated or does not pass barium in 2 to 3 days.

→

J. Studies of the Gastrointestinal Tract (continued)

Name	Description	NURSING INTERVENTION Preprocedure	NURSING INTERVENTION Postprocedure
Lower gastrointestinal (LGI) series (barium enema)	A barium enema is given, and x-ray films are taken of the large intestine.	A laxative may be given the night before the test. Liquids are restricted after midnight before the test. Enemas or suppositories are given on the morning of the test to clean the bowel. The barium enema creates a feeling of fullness, and the client will feel the urge to defecate. Test usually lasts 30 to 45 minutes. There may be some cramping. Special tubes with balloons are often used to help the client retain the barium.	Provide a rest period afterward; the procedure is fatiguing. Encourage fluids to prevent constipation. Observe stool for passage of barium, and assess regularity of bowel movements. Notify physician if barium does not pass in 2 to 3 days. An enema may be required if client does not pass all the barium.

The client is asked to assume various positions (eg, left lateral, then right lateral). Client will probably pass the barium at the x-ray department.

K. STUDIES OF THE GALLBLADDER AND BILE DUCTS

Name	Description	NURSING INTERVENTION Preprocedure	NURSING INTERVENTION Postprocedure
Cholecystography (oral cholecystography)	X-ray films are taken of the gallbladder after a contrast dye has been given orally.	A fat-free supper is given the evening before. Check for allergy to the contrast dye, which contains iodine. A laxative may be given the evening before, or an enema the morning of the test. Six or more contrast pills (eg, Telepaque) are given in 5-minute intervals the evening before the test, each with 4 to 6 oz. water. The client fasts from midnight the evening before but may drink water.	Provide a rest period. Have client resume a regular diet. Provide a snack if the client is hungry. Assess allergy to the contrast dye.

Intravenous cholangiography	X-ray films are taken of the bile ducts after dye has been administered intravenously.	The client fasts from midnight the evening before the test but may drink water. The bowel is cleaned with a laxative the evening before or with an enema the morning of the test. Check for allergy to iodine contained in the dye. Explain that iodine dye is given intravenously in the x-ray department. A test for allergy is given in the arm before the test.	Explain that (a) a fatty drink may be given during the test, (b) no discomfort is usually felt, and (c) the procedure lasts about 30 to 45 minutes.	Assess for allergy to the dye. Observe IV site for bleeding, tenderness.

→

K. Studies of the Gallbladder and Bile Ducts *(continued)*

Name	Description	NURSING INTERVENTION Preprocedure	NURSING INTERVENTION Postprocedure
Percutaneous transhepatic cholangiography	A needle is inserted through the abdominal wall into the biliary radicle, and a contrast agent is injected. Test distinguishes obstructive from nonobstructive jaundice.	Study lasts 3 to 4 hours. See preparation for intravenous cholangiography. Explain that procedure lasts about 30 minutes.	Monitor vital signs q15 minutes for 1 hour, q30 minutes for 4 hours, and then q4h until client is stable. Encourage bed rest. Position client on right side to place pressure on the puncture site to prevent bleeding.
Postoperative cholangiography	Dye is injected through the T-tube; x-ray films are taken and fluoroscopy is done to determine whether the common bile duct is unobstructed.	See preparation for intravenous cholangiography.	Monitor puncture site for bleeding. If T-tube is in place, clamp or attach to drainage as ordered. If T-tube is removed, apply sterile dressing.

L. RADIOGRAPHIC STUDIES: INTRAVENOUS PYELOGRAPHY, ANGIOGRAPHY, MYELOGRAPHY

Name	Description	NURSING INTERVENTION Preprocedure	NURSING INTERVENTION Postprocedure
Intravenous pyelography or urography (IVP, IVU)	An intravenous injection of radiopaque material is given to examine the kidneys and ureters.	A strong laxative (eg, castor oil) is given in the afternoon before the test to clear the bowel of fecal material, which can obstruct the view of the urinary structures. The client fasts from midnight prior to the test. Check for allergy to iodine. Explain that (a) an intravenous injection will be administered in the x-ray department and (b) the procedure lasts about 1 hour.	Encourage fluid intake. The client resumes a regular diet. Provide for rest; the laxative and fasting can cause weakness. Observe for reactions to the radiopaque dye.

→

L. Radiographic Studies: Intravenous Pyelography, Angiography, Myelography *(continued)*

Name	Description	NURSING INTERVENTION Preprocedure	NURSING INTERVENTION Postprocedure
Angiography, for example, cerebral angiography (vascular system of the brain), coronary arteriography (coronary arteries), renal angiography (vascular system of the kidneys), pulmonary angiography (vascular system of the lungs)	A radiopaque material is injected into an artery or vein to examine portions of the vascular system.	For some of these procedures, a catheter may be inserted into an artery or vein prior to the injection of radiopaque material. Before some procedures, the client is given a sedative. The client fasts from midnight prior to the test. A strong laxative may be given the evening before certain tests (eg, renal arteriography). Client is tested for allergy to iodine. The time needed for these procedures varies. Some may take up to 3 hours.	Bed rest is generally maintained for up to 12 hours. Monitor the client's radial pulse, respirations, and blood pressure q 15 to 30 minutes until they stabilize. Monitor peripheral pulses distal to the injection site. Observe the injection site for bleeding, and swelling. Apply cold pack to prevent swelling. Determine any discomfort experienced by the client.

| Myelography | A contrast material is injected into the subarachnoid space, and X-ray films are taken of the spinal cord, nerve roots, and vertebrae. | Fasting may be required from midnight prior to the test. The client may be given a sedative prior to the procedure. Explain that (a) a radiopaque oil dye is injected via a lumbar puncture in the X-ray department; (b) the client will assume various positions (eg, lateral for a lumbar puncture, then prone, and then tilted on X-ray table equipped with shoulder and foot supports); and (c) client may feel some pain when the oil is removed. The pain is due to irritation of the nerve roots. The procedure may last about 2 hours. | The client is generally positioned flat in bed for 24 hours to minimize headache and/or nausea; however, client may be positioned with the head elevated above the level of the spine if the dye has not been completely removed. This prevents the dye from moving to the head and causing an inflammation of the meninges (meningitis). Monitor vital signs and neurologic status (eg, complaints of numbness, pain, or tingling in the extremities; muscle weakness). Monitor urinary output. |

M. KEY INFORMATION ABOUT VITAMINS

Fat-Soluble Vitamins	RDA for Healthy Adults Ages 19 to 50	Major Dietary Sources	Major Functions	Signs of Severe, Prolonged Deficiency	Signs of Extreme Excess
A	Females: 800 RE Males: 1000 RE	Fat-containing and fortified dairy products; liver; provitamin carotene in orange and deep green fruits and vegetables	Vitamin A is a component of rhodopsin; carotenoids can serve as antioxidants; retinoic acid affects gene expression; still under intense study	Night blindness; keratinization of epithelial tissues, including the cornea of the eye (xerophthalmia), causing permanent blindness; dry, scaling skin; increased susceptibility to infection	*Preformed vitamin A:* damage to liver; bone; headache; irritability; vomiting; hair loss; blurred vision *13–cis retinoic acid:* some fetal defects *Carotenoids:* yellowed skin

D	< 25 years: 10 μg > 25 years: 5 μg	Fortified and full-fat dairy products, egg yolk (diet often not as important as sunlight exposure)	Promotes absorption and use of calcium and phosphorus	Rickets (bone deformities) in children; osteomalacia (bone softening) in adults	Calcium deposition in tissues leading to cerebral, CV, and kidney damage
E	Females: 8 α-tocopherol equivalents Males: 10 α-tocopherol equivalents	Vegetable oils and their products; nuts, seeds	Antioxidant to prevent cell membrane damage; still under intense study	Possible anemia and neurologic effects	Generally nontoxic, but at least one type of intravenous infusion led to some fatalities in premature infants; may worsen clotting defect in vitamin K deficiency

→

M. Key Information About Vitamins *(continued)*

Fat-Soluble Vitamins	RDA for Healthy Adults Ages 19 to 50	Major Dietary Sources	Major Functions	Signs of Severe, Prolonged Deficiency	Signs of Extreme Excess
K	Females: <25: 60 μg >25: 65 μg Males: <25: 70 μg >25: 80 μg	Green vegetables; tea	Aids in formation of certain proteins, especially those for blood clotting	Defective blood coagulation causing severe bleeding on injury	Liver damage and anemia from high doses of the synthetic form menadione
Water-Soluble Vitamins					
Thiamin (B^1)	Females: 1.1 mg Males: 1.5 mg	Pork, legumes, peanuts, enriched or whole-grain products	Coenzyme used in energy metabolism	Nerve changes, sometimes edema, heart failure; beriberi	Generally nontoxic, but repeated injections may cause shock reaction

Vitamin	RDA	Sources	Function	Deficiency Symptoms	Toxicity Symptoms
Riboflavin (B^2)	Females: 1.3 mg Males: 1.7 mg	Dairy products, meats, eggs, enriched grain products, green leafy vegetables	Coenzyme used in energy metabolism	Skin lesions	Generally nontoxic
Niacin	Females: 15 niacin equivalents Males: 19 niacin equivalents	Nuts, meats; provitamin tryptophan in most proteins	Coenzyme used in energy metabolism	Pellagra (multiple vitamin deficiencies including niacin)	Flushing of face, neck, hands; potential liver damage
B^6	Females: 1.6 mg Males: 2.0 mg	High-protein foods in general	Coenzyme used in amino acid metabolism	Nervous, skin, and muscular disorders; anemia	Unstable gait, numb feet, poor coordination
Folic acid	Females: 180 μg Males: 200 μg	Green vegetables, orange juice, nuts, legumes, grain products	Coenzyme used in DNA and RNA metabolism; single carbon utilization	Megaloblastic anemia (large, immature red blood cells); GI disturbances	Masks vitamin B^{12} deficiency, interferes with drugs to control epilepsy

→

M. Key Information About Vitamins (continued)

Water-Soluble Vitamins	RDA for Healthy Adults Ages 19 to 50	Major Dietary Sources	Major Functions	Signs of Severe, Prolonged Deficiency	Signs of Extreme Excess
B^{12}	2 μg	Animal products	Coenzyme used in DNA and RNA metabolism; single carbon utilization	Megaloblastic anemia; pernicious anemia when due to inadequate intrinsic factor; nervous system damage	Thought to be nontoxic
Pantothenic acid	4 to 7 mg*	Animal products and whole grains; widely distributed in foods	Coenzyme used in energy metabolism	Fatigue, numbness, and tingling of hands and feet	Generally nontoxic; occasionally causes diarrhea

	30 to 100 μg*	Widely distributed in foods	Coenzyme used in energy metabolism	Scaly dermatitis	Thought to be nontoxic
Biotin					
C (ascorbic acid)	60 mg	Fruits and vegetables, especially broccoli, cabbage, cantaloupe, cauliflower, citrus fruits, green pepper, kiwi fruit, strawberries	Functions in synthesis of collagen; is an antioxidant; aids in detoxification; improves iron absorption; still under intense study	Scurvy; petechiae (minute hemorrhages around hair follicles); weakness; delayed wound healing; impaired immune response	GI upsets, confounds certain lab tests

*Estimated Safe and Adequate Daily Dietary Intake in 1989 RDAs.

Sources: RDA Subcommittee. 1989. *Recommended dietary allowances.* Washington DC: National Academy Press. Shils, M.E. and V.R. Young, 1988. *Modern Nutrition in Health and Disease.* Philadelphia: Lea & Febiger.

N. KEY INFORMATION ABOUT MINERALS

Major Mineral	RDA for Healthy Adults Ages 19 to 50	Major Dietary Sources	Major Functions	Signs of Severe, Prolonged Deficiency	Signs of Extreme Excess
Calcium	1200 mg for ages 19 to 24; 800 mg for 25 and older	Milk, cheese, dark green vegetables, legumes	Bone and tooth formation; blood clotting; nerve transmission	Stunted growth; perhaps less bone mass	Depressed absorption of some other minerals; perhaps kidney damage
Phosphorus	1200 mg for ages 19 to 24; 800 mg for 25 and older	Milk, cheese, meat, poultry, whole grains	Bone and tooth formation; acid-base balance; component of coenzymes	Weakness; demineralization of bone	Depressed absorption of some minerals
Magnesium	Females: 280 mg Males: 350 mg	Whole grains, green leafy vegetables	Component of enzymes	Neurologic disturbances	Neurologic disturbances

				(Related to protein deficiency)	Excess
Sulfur	(Provided by sulfur amino acids)	Sulfur amino acids in dietary proteins	Component of cartilage, tendons, and proteins	(Related to protein deficiency)	Excess sulfur-containing amino acid intake leads to poor growth; liver damage
Sodium	*	Salt, soy sauce, cured meats, pickles, canned soups, processed cheese	Body water balance; nerve function	Muscle cramps; reduced appetite	High blood pressure in genetically predisposed individuals
Potassium	*	Meats, milk, many fruits and vegetables, whole grains	Body water balance; nerve function	Muscular weakness; paralysis	Muscular weakness; cardiac arrest
Chloride	*	Same as for sodium	Plays a role in acid-base balance; formation of gastric juice	Muscle cramps; reduced appetite; poor growth	High blood pressure in genetically predisposed individuals

N. Key Information About Trace Minerals

Trace Mineral	RDA for Healthy Adults Ages 19 to 50	Major Dietary Sources	Major Functions	Signs of Severe, Prolonged Deficiency	Signs of Extreme Excess
Iron	Females: 15 mg Males: 10 mg	Meats, eggs, legumes, whole grains, green leafy vegetables	Components of hemoglobin, myoglobin, and enzymes	Iron deficiency anemia, weakness, impaired immune function	*Acute:* shock, death; *Chronic:* liver damage, cardiac failure
Iodine	150 μg	Fish and shellfish; dairy products; iodized salt, some breads	Component of thyroid hormones	Goiter (enlarged thyroid)	Iodide goiter
Fluoride	1.5 to 4 mg†	Drinking water, tea, seafood	Maintenance of tooth (and maybe bone) structure	Higher frequency of tooth decay	*Acute:* GI distress *Chronic:* mottling of teeth; skeletal deformation

			Component of	Deficiency	Toxicity
Zinc	Females: 12 mg Males: 15 mg	Meats, seafood, whole grains	Component of enzymes	Growth failure; scaly dermatitis; reproductive failure; impaired immune function	*Acute:* nausea; vomiting; diarrhea *Chronic:* adversely affects copper metabolism and immune function; anemia
Selenium	Females: 55 μg Males: 70 μg	Seafood, meats, whole grains	Component of enzymes; functions in close association with vitamin E	Muscle pain; maybe heart muscle deterioration	Nausea and vomiting; hair and nail loss
Copper	1.5 to 3 mg[†]	Seafood, nuts, legumes, organ meats	Component of enzymes	Anemia; bone and cardiovascular changes	Nausea; liver damage

→

N. Key Information About Trace Minerals (continued)

Trace Mineral	RDA for Healthy Adults Ages 19 to 50	Major Dietary Sources	Major Functions	Signs of Severe, Prolonged Deficiency	Signs of Extreme Excess
Cobalt	(Required as vitamin B[12])*	Animal products	Component of vitamin B[12]	Not reported except as vitamin B[12] deficiency	With alcohol: heart failure
Chromium	50 to 200 µg[†]	Brewer's yeast, liver, seafood, meat, some vegetables	Involved in glucose and energy metabolism	Impaired glucose metabolism	Lung and kidney damage (occupational exposures only)
Manganese	2 to 5 mg[†]	Nuts, whole grains, vegetables and fruits, tea	Component of enzymes	Abnormal bone and cartilage	Central nervous system damage (occupational exposures)

| Molybdenum | 75 to 250 μg† | Legumes, cereals, some vegetables | Component of enzymes | Disorder in nitrogen excretion | Inhibition of enzymes; adversely affects copper metabolism |

*No formal recommendation
†Estimated safe and adequate daily dietary intake.

References

Moore, M. 1997. *Mosby's Pocket Guide Series to Nutritional Care*. St Louis: Mosby.

RDA Subcommittee. 1989. *Recommended Dietary Allowances*. Washington, DC: National Academy Press.

Williams, S. 1997. *Nutrition and Diet Therapy*. St Louis: Mosby.

O. INFECTION CONTROL STRATEGIES

- Use strict aseptic technique when performing any invasive procedure (for example, inserting an intravenous needle or catheter, suctioning an airway, and inserting a urinary catheter) and when changing surgical dressings. See Chapters 33, 35, 46, 47, and 48.

- Handle needles and syringes carefully to avoid needle prick injuries. See Chapter 33.

- Change intravenous tubing and solution containers according to hospital policy (for example, every 48 to 72 hours). See Chapter 48.

- Check all sterile supplies for expiration date and intact packaging.

- Prevent urinary infections by maintaining a closed urinary drainage system with a downhill flow of urine; do not irrigate a catheter unless ordered to do so; provide regular catheter care; clean the perineal area with soap and water; and keep the drainage bag and spout off the floor. See Chapter 46.

- Implement measures to prevent impaired skin integrity (see Chapter 34) and to prevent accumulation of secretions in the lungs (for example, encourage the client to move, cough, and breathe deeply at least every 2 hours).

Steps to Follow After Exposure to Bloodborne Pathogens

- For a puncture/laceration:

  a. Encourage bleeding.

  b. Wash/clean the area with soap and water.

  c. Initiate first-aid and seek treatment if indicated.

- For a mucous membrane exposure (eyes, nose, mouth), saline or water flush for 5–10 minutes.

- Report the incident immediately to appropriate personnel within the agency.

- Complete an injury report.

- Seek appropriate evaluation and follow-up. This includes the following:

  a. Identification and documentation of the source individual when feasible and legal

  b. Testing of the source individual's blood when feasible and consent is given

  c. Making results of the test available to the source individual's health care provider

  d. Testing of blood of exposed health care provider (with consent)

  e. Post exposure prophylaxis, if medically indicated (eg, hepatitis B vaccine for HBV, or recommended agents for HIV)

  f. Medical counseling regarding personal risk of infection or risk of infecting others

P. RECOMMENDED CHILDHOOD IMMUNIZATION SCHEDULE—UNITED STATES

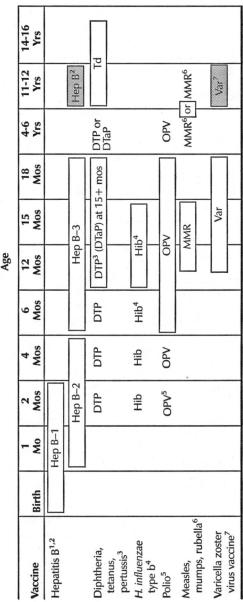

Age

Vaccine	Birth	1 Mo	2 Mos	4 Mos	6 Mos	12 Mos	15 Mos	18 Mos	4-6 Yrs	11-12 Yrs	14-16 Yrs
Hepatitis B[1,2]	Hep B-1	Hep B-1 / Hep B-2	Hep B-2		Hep B-3	Hep B-3	Hep B-3	Hep B-3		Hep B[2]	
Diphtheria, tetanus, pertussis[3]			DTP	DTP	DTP	DTP[3] (DTaP) at 15+ mos	DTP[3] (DTaP) at 15+ mos	DTP[3] (DTaP) at 15+ mos	DTP or DTaP	Td	Td
H. influenzae type b[4]			Hib	Hib	Hib[4]	Hib[4]	Hib[4]				
Polio[5]			OPV[5]	OPV	OPV	OPV	OPV	OPV	OPV		
Measles, mumps, rubella[6]						MMR	MMR		MMR[6] or	MMR[6]	
Varicella zoster virus vaccine[7]						Var	Var	Var		Var[7]	

Source: From *Pediatrics* 97(1):143. 1996

Approved by the Advisory Committee on Immunization Practices (ACIP), the American Academy of Family Physicians (AAFP).

Vaccines are listed under the routinely recommended ages.
Bars indicate range of acceptable ages for vaccination.
Shaded bars indicate *catch-up vaccination:* at 11–12 years of age, hepatitis B vaccine should be administered to children not previously vaccinated, and Varicella Zoster Virus vaccine should be administered to children not previously vaccinated who lack a reliable history of chickenpox. A decision to use the new rotavirus vaccine (RV) should be made together by the parent and pediatrician.

[1]*Infants born to HBsAg-negative mothers* should receive 2.5 μg of Merck vaccine (Recombivax HB) or 10 μg of SmithKline Beecham (SB) vaccine (Energix-B). The 2nd dose should be administered ≤ 1 mo after the 1st dose.

Infants born to HBsAg-positive mothers should receive 0.5ml. Hepatitis B Immune Globulin (HBIG) within 12 hr of birth, and either 5 μg of Merck vaccine (Recombivax HB) or 10 μg of SB vaccine (Energix-B) at a separate site. The 2nd dose is recommended at 1–2 mos of age and the 3rd dose at 6 mos of age.

Infants born to mothers whose HBsAg status is unknown should receive either 5 μg of Merck vaccine (Recombivax HB) or 10 μg of SB vaccine (Energix-B) within 12 hr of birth. The 2nd dose of vaccine is recommended at 1 mo of age and the 3rd dose at 6 mos of age.

[2]Adolescents who have not previously received 3 doses of hepatitis B vaccine should initiate or complete the series at the 11–12 year-old visit. The 2nd dose should be administered at least 1 mo after the 1st dose and the 3rd dose should be administered at least 4 mos after the 1st dose and at least 2 mos after the 2nd dose.

[3]DTP4 may be administered at 12 mos of age, if at least 6 mos have elapsed since DTP3. DTaP (diphtheria and tetanus toxoids and acellular pertussis vaccine is licensed for the 4th and/or 5th vaccine dose(s) for children aged ≤ 15 mos and may be preferred for these doses in this age group. Td (tetanus and diphtheria toxoids, adsorbed, for adult use) is recommended at 11–12 years of age if at least 5 years have elapsed since the last dose of DTP, DTaP, or DT.

[4]Three *H. influenzae* type b (Hib) conjugate vaccines are licensed for infant use. If PRP-OMP (Pedvax HIB [Merck]) is administered at 2 and 4 mos of age, a dose at 6 mos is not required. After completing the primary series, any HIB conjugate vaccine may be used as a booster.

[5]Oral poliovirus vaccine (OPV) is recommended for routine infant vaccination. Inactivated poliovirus vaccine (IPV) is recommended for persons with a congenital or acquired immune deficiency disease or an altered immune status as a result of disease or immunosuppressive therapy, as well as their household contacts, and is an acceptable alternative for other persons. The primary 3-dose series for IPV should be given with a minimum interval of 4 wks between the 1st and 2nd doses and 6 mos between the 2nd and 3rd doses.

[6]The 2nd dose of MMR is routinely recommended at 4–6 yrs of age or at 11–12 yrs of age, but may be administered at any visit, provided at least 1 mo has elapsed since receipt of the 1st dose.

[7]Varicella zoster virus vaccine (Var) can be administered to susceptible children any time after 12 months of age. Unvaccinated children who lack a reliable history of chickenpox should be vaccinated at the 11–12 year-old visit.

Q. IMMUNIZATION FOR HIGH-RISK ADULTS

Vaccine*	High-Risk Groups
Diphtheria-tetanus	Adults who have not been immunized during the past 10 years, and after trauma and puncture wounds
Pneumococcal infections	People 65 years and older, residents in nursing homes and prisons, adults who have chronic medical problems (eg, cardio-vascular or respiratory disease)
Hepatitis B	All health care workers, hemophiliac clients, hemodialysis clients, intravenous drug users, immigrants from countries where there is endemic disease, people who are sexually active with multiple partners
Influenza	Health care workers, older people residing in nursing homes, adults who have chronic diseases (eg, respiratory illnesses, diabetes, cardiovascular problems)
Measles-mumps-rubella (MMR)	Adults who have not been immunized, especially women of childbearing age, healthcare workers, adults born before 1956 and immunized before 12 months of age

*Determine the recommended immunization for a specific country or jurisdiction when traveling.

UNIT 2

Assessment and Diagnosis

A. Nursing Health History
B. Methods of Examining
C. Vital Signs
D. Physical Health Examination
E. NANDA Nursing Diagnoses

A. NURSING HEALTH HISTORY

The nursing health history is the first part of the assessment of the client's health status. Through this structured interview, you collect specific health data and obtain a detailed health record of the client. The client is the primary source of information.

You may also consult other sources for information about the client's health, including the medical record if available, and consultations with members of the health care team, family members, or significant others. It is important to be systematic in your approach and document your findings.

Before starting the interview, be sure to introduce yourself and state your purpose for collecting data. Establish rapport to put the client at ease and facilitate the interview process.

Biographic Data
- Start your interview by asking for biographic data such as age, marital status, occupation, religious orientation, primary language spoken, usual source of medical care, and insurance information.

Chief Concern (Complaint)
- Next, ask the reason for this visit or hospitalization. Ask questions such as, "What brought you

to the hospital?" or "What is troubling you?" Answers to these questions will help you determine the chief concern.

History of Present Illness

Usual Health Status

- How would you describe your health up until this time?

Chronologic Story

- When did symptoms start?
- Was the onset sudden or gradual?
- How often does the problem occur?
- Where is the exact location of distress?
- Has the problem occurred before?
- Were home or other remedies used for the problem?
- What activity were you involved in when the problem occurred?
- What factors aggravate or alleviate the problem?

Relevant Family History

- Do any family members have a similar health problem?

Disability Assessment

- Do any family members have a similar health problem?

Past History

- What childhood illnesses have you had? Have you been immunized? When did you last have a tetanus shot?

- Do you have any allergies? What type?

- Have you had any accidents or injuries requiring medical attention? Note dates and treatment received. Are there any lasting effects?

- Have you ever been hospitalized? Where? When? Why?

- Are you currently taking any prescription or over-the-counter medications on a regular basis? Note all medications, how long the client has been taking them, and why.

Family History of Illness

- What is the health of family members? Are there histories of cancer, hypertension, diabetes, or heart disease (and so on)? This information reveals risk factors for the client.

Lifestyle

- Do you use tobacco, alcohol, illicit or recreational drugs? Note frequency and amounts. What is your diet? Sleep/rest patterns? Activities of daily living? Recreation/hobbies?

Social Data

- Do you have friends and family? If so, what support do they, or can they, provide?

- With which cultural or ethnic group(s) are you affiliated? Do not make assumptions based on race, dress, or language.

- What is your educational level?

- What is your occupational history?

- How would you describe your financial status?

- What are your home and neighborhood conditions?

Psychologic Data

- How does the client appear? Happy? Sad? Is body language congruent to what the client is saying? Is the client dressed appropriately? Clean? Unkempt?

- How do you feel?

- What are your major stressors?

- What do you normally do to cope with a serious problem?

- What is your communication style?

Review of Systems

The goal of the review of systems is to gather subjective data from the client on each of the major body systems. See the checklist below.

- *General health*. Weight loss, weakness, feelings of fatigue, mood changes, night sweats, or bleeding tendencies?

- *Skin*. Skin diseases such as eczema, psoriasis, acne; change in pigmentation; tendency toward bruising; excessive dryness or moisture; jaundice; itching, rashes, hives; change in color or size of moles; or open sores that are slow to heal?

- *Hair.* Itchy scalp, loss of hair, excessive body hair? Does the client wear a wig?

- *Nails.* Color changes, biting, clubbing, splitting?

- *Head.* Frequent or severe headaches, fainting, dizziness, accident resulting in unconsciousness?

- *Eyes.* Difficulty seeing, eye infection, eye pain, excessive tearing, double vision, blurring, sensitivity to light, cataracts, itching, spots in front of eyes? Does the client wear glasses (for near or far vision) or contact lenses? When was the client's last eye examination?

- *Ears.* Any infection, loss of hearing, pain, discharge, ringing in the ears? Does the client wear a hearing aid?

- *Nose.* Frequent colds, nosebleeds, allergies, pain, tenderness, postnasal drip?

- *Mouth and throat.* Sore gums; bleeding gums; sores, lumps or white spots on mouth, lips or tongue; toothaches, cavities, difficulty swallowing; voice change or hoarseness? Does the client wear dentures (upper, lower, partial)? When was the client's last dental appointment?

- *Neck.* Pain, swelling, stiffness, limited movement, swollen glands?

- *Breasts.* Nipple discharge, scaling or cracks around nipples, dimples, lumps, pattern of breast self-examination? Last mammogram?

- *Respiratory system.* Chest pain; cough; shortness of breath; wheezing; coughing up blood; lung disease such as tuberculosis, emphysema, asthma, bronchitis? Has the client ever had a chest x-ray? When? Results?

- *Cardiovascular system.* Heart disease, palpitations, heart murmur, high blood pressure, anemia, varicose veins, leg swelling or ulcer?

- *Gastrointestinal system.* Nausea, vomiting, loss of appetite, indigestion, heartburn, bright blood in stools, tarry-black stools, diarrhea, constipation, abdominal pain, excessive gas, hemorrhoids, rectal pain, colostomy, ileostomy?

- *Genitourinary system.* Frequency, dribbling, urgency, urination at night, difficulty starting stream, blood in urine, incontinence, pain or burning upon urination, urinary tract infection, ureterostomy, sexually transmitted disease such as gonorrhea or syphilis?

  Females: Age of menarche, last menstrual period (LMP), duration, amount of flow, regularity of cycle? Any problems with painful menstruation, bleeding between periods, pain during intercourse, vaginal discharge, vaginal itching, vaginal infection?

  Males: Penile discharge, swelling, masses or lesions, difficulty in sexual functioning?

- *Musculoskeletal system.* Muscular pain, swelling, or weakness; joint swelling, soreness, or stiffness; leg cramps; bone defects?

- *Neurologic system.* Difficulty walking; unconsciousness; seizures; tremors; paralysis; numbness, tingling or burning sensations in any body part; weakness on one side of body; speech problems; loss of memory; disorientation; forgetfulness; unclear thinking; changes in emotional state?

- *Endocrine system.* History of goiter; heat or cold intolerance; diabetes; excessive thirst; excessive eating?

B. METHODS OF EXAMINING

There are four primary techniques you will use in the physical examination: inspection, palpation, percussion, and auscultation.

Inspection

Inspection, or visual examination, should be done systematically, with sufficient light.

Palpation

Palpation is the use of the sense of touch to determine texture, temperature, vibration, position, size, consistency, mobility, distention, pulse rates, and tenderness or pain.

Percussion

In percussion, the body surface is struck to elicit sounds that can be heard or vibrations that can be felt.

Percussion is used to determine the size and shape of the internal organs by establishing their borders. It indicates whether tissue is fluid-filled, air-filled, or solid. Percussion elicits five types of sounds:

- Flatness (dull)—bone and muscle

- Dullness (thudlike)—liver, spleen, heart

- Resonance (hollow)—air-filled lung

- Hyperresonance (booming)—emphysematous lung

- Tympany (drumlike)—air-filled stomach

There are two types of percussion methods: direct/immediate and indirect/mediate.

Direct/Immediate Percussion

- Strike the area to be percussed with two or more fingers, using the pads of the fingers only.

- Use rapid wrist movements.

Indirect/Mediate Percussion

- Place the middle finger of your nondominant hand firmly on the skin of the area to be percussed. (Use only the distal phalanx and joint of the finger.)

- Using the flexed middle finger of the dominant hand, strike the middle finger of the nondominant hand. Be sure to use rapid wrist movements.

Auscultation

Auscultation is the process of listening to sounds produced within the body. The use of an unaided ear is the direct method of auscultation. The use of a stethoscope is considered an indirect method. Auscultated sounds are described according to the following:

- Pitch—frequency of vibrations

- Intensity—loudness or softness

- Duration—length of the sound

- Quality—subjective description of the sound

C. VITAL SIGNS

Vital signs are obtained to monitor the functions of the body. The temperature, pulse, respiratory rate, and blood pressure measurements indicate how the body is functioning or responding to medications or treatments. Refer to Chapter 28 of *Fundamentals of Nursing* for a thorough discussion of vital signs.

Temperature

Temperature is a measurement of the balance between heat produced by the body and heat lost from the body. A fever results from inadequate heat loss; a low temperature, from excessive heat loss. When measured orally, adult temperature is 36.7C to 37C. Temperatures can be taken via the following methods:

- *Oral*—Leave in place for 3 to 5 minutes to register, or for the length of time recommended by the agency. If the client is too young or too confused to cooperate, use another means of measuring temperature.

- *Rectal*—Leave in place approximately 2 minutes or for the length of time recommended by the agency. Use a lubricant. Do not use the rectal method if client has rectal disease or convulsions. Be sure to hold a child firmly.

- *Axillary*—Leave in place approximately 9 minutes for adults and 5 minutes for children, or according to agency protocol.

Electronic thermometers can be used in any of these routes. Leave the thermometer in place until the device beeps and flashes the value.

Pulse

The pulse is a wave of blood created by contraction of the heart's left ventricle. The nine sites where pulses are commonly taken are (1) temporal, (2) carotid, (3) apical, (4) brachial, (5) radial (most common), (6) femoral, (7) popliteal, (8) posterior tibial, and (9) pedal. See the figure on page 113 for pulse sites.

To take a client's pulse, take the following steps:

- Before taking the pulse, ensure that the client is at rest. If the client has been active, wait 10 to 15 minutes.

- Use your index and middle fingers to palpate all pulse sites, except for the apex of the heart, where a stethoscope is required.

- Note rate, rhythm, volume, arterial wall elasticity, presence of bilateral equality, and intensity.

- Count irregular pulses a full 60 seconds.

Respirations

When assessing respirations, note the rate (breaths per minute), depth (normal, deep, or shallow), rhythm (regularity), and quality (effort required to breathe, and the sound of the respirations). Whenever possible, assess respirations when the client is

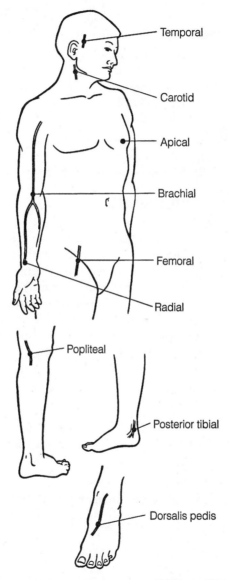

Temporal

Carotid

Apical

Brachial

Femoral

Radial

Popliteal

Posterior tibial

Dorsalis pedis

unaware that you are doing so. Use the following methods to assess respirations:

- While you are standing at the bedside, ask the client to place the arm farthest away from you across the chest, if possible. The arm will rise and fall as the client breathes, making it easier to count respirations.

- After assessing the pulse, continue holding the wrist. Count the respiratory rate and observe the depth, rhythm, and quality of respirations.

Blood Pressure

Blood pressure is a measure of the pressure the blood exerts as it flows through the arteries. The systolic pressure (the top number) measures the amount of pressure during contraction of the ventricles, and the diastolic pressure (the bottom number) is the measure of the pressure in the ventricles when they are at rest. Blood pressures can be taken on the arm or on the thigh. Points to remember include the following:

- Be sure the cuff is of adequate size. For the obese client, use a large cuff or thigh cuff. The cuff should be wide enough to cover 2/3 of the upper arm.

- Make sure the client is calm and has not smoked or exercised within 30 minutes of the measurement.

- Inspect the arm or thigh before placing the cuff. Do not use an extremity that has an IV line, a shunt in place, or is injured.

D. PHYSICAL HEALTH EXAMINATION

A complete health assessment is generally conducted from the head to the toes; however, the procedure can vary in many ways according to the age of the individual, the severity of the illness, the preferences of the nurse, and the agency's priorities and procedures. Regardless of what procedure is used, the client's energy and time need to be considered. The health assessment is therefore conducted in a systematic and efficient manner that requires the fewest position changes for the client. Refer to Chapter 29 of *Fundamentals of Nursing* for a thorough discussion of the physical health examination.

Frequently, nurses assess a specific body area instead of the entire body. These specific assessments are made in relation to client complaints, the nurse's own observation of the problem, the client's presenting problem, nursing interventions provided, and medical therapies.

While you are assessing the client, don't be afraid to talk and ask questions. Conversation puts the client at ease and gives you valuable subjective information.

Preparing the Client

Most people need an explanation of the physical health examination. Explain when and where the examination will take place, why it is necessary, who will conduct it, and what will happen during the examination. Also, inform the client of any special circumstances—for instance, the need to go to a different room or assume a special position—and tell the client that appropriate draping will be provided so that the body will not be unnecessarily exposed.

Most clients should empty the bladder before the examination. Doing so helps them feel more relaxed and facilitates palpation of the abdomen and pubic area. Because an empty rectum facilitates rectal examination, encourage the client to defecate before a complete physical examination. If a urinalysis is required, urine should be collected in a container for that purpose.

In conducting a physical examination, you will use the four methods of assessment: inspection, palpation, percussion, and auscultation. You will also be collecting subjective data, which is what the client tells you (such as, "I feel dizzy"), and objective data, which is what you can see, quantify, touch, or smell (for example, BP of 80/50). For example, low blood pressure is the objective finding for the subjective assessment of dizziness.

Before you start, be sure to do the following:

- Collect your equipment.

- Explain to the client what you will be doing and approximately how long it will take to complete the examination. Establishing rapport with the client will make for a more relaxed examination for both of you.

- Wash your hands. Follow universal precautions throughout.

- Ensure that the client's privacy is protected. Draw the curtain if the room is semi-private.

Assessing the Client
General Survey
Appearance
- Observe body build, height, and weight in relation to the client's age, lifestyle, and health.

- Observe the client's posture and gait, standing, sitting, and walking.

- Observe the client's overall hygiene and grooming. Relate these to the person's activities prior to the assessment.

- Note body and breath odor in relation to activity level.

- Observe for signs of distress in posture (eg, bending over because of abdominal pain) or facial expressions (eg, wincing or labored breathing).

- Note obvious signs of health or illness (eg, in skin color or breathing).

Mental Status
- Assess the client's attitude.

- Note the client's affect/mood; assess the appropriateness of the client's responses.

- Listen for quantity of speech (amount and pace), quality (loudness, clarity, inflection), and organization (coherence of thought, overgeneralization, vagueness).

- Listen for relevance and organization of thoughts.

The Integument
Skin
- Inspect skin color (best assessed under natural lighting and on areas not exposed to the sun).

- Inspect uniformity of skin color.

- Assess edema, if present (eg, location, color, temperature, shape, and the degree to which the skin remains indented or pitted when pressed by a finger).

- Inspect, palpate, and describe skin lesions. Palpate lesions to determine shape and texture. Describe lesions according to location, type or structure, color, distribution, and configuration.

- Observe and palpate skin moisture.

- Palpate skin temperature. Compare the two feet and two hands using the backs of your fingers.

- Note skin turgor (fullness or elasticity) by lifting and pinching the skin on an extremity.

Hair
- Inspect the distribution of growth over the scalp.

- Inspect hair thickness or thinness.

- Inspect hair texture and oiliness.

- Note the presence of infections or infestations by parting the hair in several areas.

- Inspect amount of body hair.

Nails

- Inspect nail plate shape to determine its curvature and angle. See the figure below and on page 120 for nail plate findings.

- Inspect nail texture.

- Inspect nail color.

- Inspect tissues surrounding nails.

- Perform blanch test to evaluate capillary refill.

About 160° (normal)

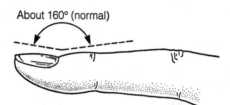

Flattened angle about 180° (early clubbing)

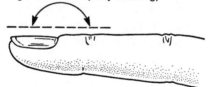

Greater than 180° angle (late clubbing)

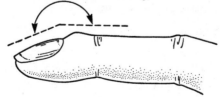

continued

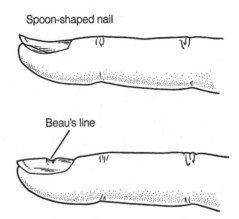

Spoon-shaped nail

Beau's line

The Head

The Skull and Face

- Inspect the skull for size, shape, and symmetry. If skull is of abnormal size, measure its circumference just above the eyebrows.

- Palpate the skull for masses, depressions, or nodules.

- Inspect the facial features (eg, symmetry of structures and of the distribution of hair).

- Inspect the eyes for edema and hollowness.

- Note symmetry of facial movements. Ask the client to elevate the eyebrows, frown, or lower the eyebrows, close the eyes tightly, puff the cheeks, and smile and show teeth.

The Eyes and Vision

External Eye Structures

- Inspect the eyebrows for hair distribution, alignment, skin quality, and movement (ask the client to raise and lower the eyebrows).

- Inspect the eyelashes for evenness of distribution and direction of the curl.

- Inspect the eyelids for surface characteristics (such as, skin quality and texture), position in relation to the cornea, ability to blink, and frequency of blinking.

- Inspect the bulbar conjunctiva (the conjunctiva lying over the sclera) for color, texture, and presence of lesions. Retract the eyelids and ask client to look up, down, and from side to side.

- Inspect the palpebral conjunctiva (the conjunctiva lining the eyelids) by everting the lower lids. Note color, texture, and presence of lesions.

- Evert upper lids if a problem is suspected.

- Inspect and palpate the lacrimal gland.

- Inspect and palpate the lacrimal sac and nasolacrimal duct.

- Inspect the corneas for clarity and texture by using a penlight at an oblique angle to the eye.

- Perform corneal sensitivity (reflex) test to determine function of the fifth (trigeminal) cranial nerve.

- Inspect the anterior chamber for transparency and depth.

- Inspect pupils for color, shape, and symmetry of size.

- Assess each pupil's direct and consensual reaction to light to determine the function of the third (oculomotor) and fourth (trochlear) cranial nerves.

- Assess each pupil's reaction to accommodation.

Visual Fields
- Assess peripheral visual fields to determine function of the retina and neuronal visual pathways to the brain and second (optic) cranial nerve.

Extraocular Muscle Tests
- Assess six ocular movements to determine eye alignment and coordination.

- Perform the cover-uncover patch test to determine eye alignment.

- Perform the corneal light reflex test to determine eye alignment.

Visual Acuity
- Assess near vision by asking the client to wear corrective lenses, unless they are used for reading only.

- Perform functional vision tests if the client is unable to see the top line of the Snellen chart.

The Ears and Hearing
Auricles
- Inspect the auricles for color, symmetry of size, and position.

- Palpate the auricles for texture, elasticity, and areas of tenderness.

External Ear Canal and Tympanic Membrane
- Using an otoscope, inspect the external ear canal for cerumen, skin lesions, pus, and blood. Inspect the tympanic membrane for color.

Gross Hearing Acuity Test
- Assess client's response to normal voice tones. If the client has difficulty hearing the normal voice, proceed with the following tests.

- Assess client's response to a whispered voice.

Tuning Fork Tests
- Perform Weber's test to assess bone conduction.

- Perform the Rinne test to compare air conduction to bone conduction.

Nose and Sinuses
- Inspect the external nose for any deviations in shape, size, symmetry, or color. Inspect for flaring or discharge from the nares.

- Lightly palpate the external nose to determine any areas of tenderness, masses, and displacements of bone and cartilage.

- Inspect the nasal cavities using a penlight or a nasal speculum.

- Determine patency of both nasal cavities.

- Palpate the maxillary and frontal sinuses for tenderness.

- Transilluminate the frontal sinuses.

- Transilluminate the maxillary sinuses.

The Mouth and Oropharynx

Lips and Buccal Mucosa

- Inspect the outer lips for symmetry of contour, color, and texture.

- Inspect and palpate the inner lips and buccal mucosa for color, moisture, texture, and the presence of lesions.

Teeth and Gums

- Inspect the teeth and gums while examining the inner lips and buccal mucosa.

- Inspect the dentures. Ask the client to remove complete or partial dentures. Inspect their condition, noting in particular broken or worn areas.

Tongue/Floor of Mouth

- Inspect the surface of the tongue for position, color, and texture by asking the client to protrude the tongue.

- Inspect tongue movement.

- Inspect the base of the tongue, the mouth floor, and the frenulum.

- Palpate the tongue and floor of the mouth for any nodules, lumps, or excoriated areas.

Salivary Glands

- Inspect salivary gland openings for any swelling or redness.

Palates and Uvula

- Inspect the hard palate and soft palate for color, shape, texture, and the presence of bony prominences.

- Inspect the uvula for position and mobility while examining the palates.

Oropharynx and Tonsils
- Inspect the oropharynx for color and texture using a tongue blade and penlight.

- Inspect the tonsils for color, discharge, and size.

- Elicit the gag reflex by pressing the posterior tongue with a tongue depressor.

The Neck
Neck Muscles
- Inspect the neck muscles for abnormal swelling or masses.

- Observe head movement. Ask the client to move the chin to the chest, to move the head back so that the chin points upward, to move the head so that the ear is moved toward the shoulder on each side, and to turn the head to the right and to the left.

- Assess muscle strength by asking the client to turn the head against the resistance of your hand. Repeat with the other side. Then ask the client to shrug the shoulders against the resistance of your hands.

Lymph Nodes
- Palpate the entire neck for presence of enlarged lymph nodes.

Trachea
- Palpate the trachea for lateral deviation.

Thyroid Gland
- Inspect the thyroid gland by standing in front of the client.

- Observe the lower half of the neck overlying the thyroid gland for symmetry and visible masses.

- Ask the client to hyperextend the head and swallow to determine thyroid and cricoid movement.

- Palpate the thyroid gland for smoothness.

- If enlargement of the gland is suspected, auscultate over the thyroid area for a bruit.

The Thorax and Lung
Posterior Thorax

- Inspect the shape and symmetry of the anterior, posterior, and lateral thorax.

- Inspect the spinal alignment for deformities.

- Palpate the posterior thorax.

- Palpate the posterior chest for respiratory excursion.

- Palpate the chest for vocal (tactile) fremitus comparing each lung side.

- Percuss the thorax. Use a systematic zigzag procedure.

- Percuss for diaphragmatic excursion during maximal inspiration and expiration.

- Auscultate the chest using the flat-disc diaphragm of the stethoscope. Ask the client to take slow, deep breaths through the mouth. Use a systematic zigzag procedure. Compare findings at each point with the corresponding point on the opposite side of the chest.

Anterior Thorax

- Inspect breathing patterns (eg, respiratory rate and rhythm).

- Inspect the costal angle and the angle at which the ribs enter the spine.

- Palpate the anterior chest for respiratory excursion and tactile fremitus.

- Percuss the anterior chest symmetrically. Begin above the clavicles in the supraclavicular space, and proceed down to the diaphragm. Compare one side of the lung to the other. Displace female breasts for proper examination.

- Auscultate the trachea.

- Auscultate the anterior chest. Use the sequence used in percussion, beginning over the bronchi between the sternum and the clavicles.

The Cardiovascular and Peripheral Vascular Systems

The Cardiovascular System

- Simultaneously inspect and palpate the precordium for the presence of abnormal pulsations, lifts, or heaves.

- Inspect and palpate the aortic, pulmonic, tricuspid, and apical areas for pulsations.

- Inspect and palpate the apical area for pulsation, noting its specific location and diameter. If displaced laterally, record the distance between the apex and the midclavicular line (MCL) in centimeters.

(text continues on page 130)

Breath Sounds

Normal

Type	Description	Location
Vesicular	Soft-intensity, low-pitched, "gentle sighing" sounds created by air moving through smaller airways (bronchioles and alveoli)	Over peripheral lung; best heard at base of lungs
Bronchovesicular	Moderate-intensity and moderate-pitched "blowing" sounds created by air moving through larger airways (bronchi)	Between the scapulae and lateral to the sternum at the first and second intercostal spaces
Bronchial (tubular)	High-pitched, loud, "harsh" sounds created by air moving through the trachea	Anteriorly over the trachea; not normally heard over lung tissue

Adventitious

Name	Description	Cause
Crackles (rales)	Fine, short, interrupted crackling sounds; alveolar rales are high-pitched; bronchial rales are lower-pitched. Sound can be simulated by rolling a lock of hair near the ear. Best heard on inspiration but can be heard on both inspiration and expiration. May not be cleared by coughing.	Air passing through fluid or mucus in any air passage
Gurgles (rhonchi)	Continuous, low-pitched, coarse, gurgling, harsh, louder sounds with a moaning or snoring quality. Best heard on expiration but can be heard on both inspiration and expiration. May be altered by coughing.	Air passing through narrowed air passages as a result of secretions, swelling, tumors
Friction rub	Superficial grating or creaking sounds heard during inspiration and expiration. Not relieved by coughing.	Rubbing together of inflamed pleural surfaces
Wheeze	Continuous, high-pitched, squeaky musical sounds. Best heard on expiration. Not usually altered by coughing.	Air passing through a constricted bronchi as a result of secretions, swelling, tumors

D. Physical Health Examination **129**

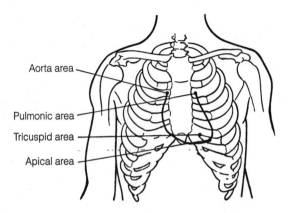

Aorta area

Pulmonic area

Tricuspid area

Apical area

- Auscultate the heart in all four anatomic sites: aortic, pulmonic, tricuspid, and apical (mitral). See the figure above.

- Inspect and palpate the epigastric area (at the base of the sternum) for abdominal aortic pulsations.

The Peripheral Vascular System

- Palpate the peripheral pulses on both sides of the client's body systematically and simultaneously to determine the symmetry of pulse volume. If you have difficulty palpating some of the peripheral pulses, use a Doppler ultrasound probe.

- Palpate the carotid arteries **using extreme caution.**

- Auscultate the carotid artery to determine the presence of a bruit.

Jugular Veins
- Inspect the jugular veins for distention while the client is in a semi-Fowler's position with the head supported on a small pillow.

Peripheral Veins

- Inspect the peripheral veins in the arms and legs for the presence or appearance of superficial veins when limbs are dependent and when limbs are elevated.

- Assess the peripheral leg veins for signs of phlebitis.

Peripheral Perfusion

- Inspect the skin of the hands and the feet for color, temperature, edema, and skin changes.

- Assess the adequacy of arterial flow if arterial insufficiency is suspected.

The Breasts and Axillae

- Use this as an opportunity to teach breast self-examination (BSE).

- Inspect and palpate the breasts of both men and women.

- Inspect the breasts for size, symmetry, and contour or shape while in a sitting position.

- Inspect the skin of the breast for localized discolorations or hyperpigmentation, retraction or dimpling, localized hypervascular areas, swelling, or edema.

- Accentuate any retraction by having the client raise the arms above the head, push the hands together with elbows fixed, and/or press the hands down on the hips.

- Inspect the areola area for size, shape, symmetry, color, surface characteristics, and any masses or lesions.

- For the male client, palpate the breasts and the axillary lymph nodes when the client is supine.

- For the female client, palpate the axillary, subclavicular, and supraclavicular lymph nodes while the client sits with the arms abducted and supported on your forearm. Use the palmar surface of all fingertips to palpate.

- Palpate the breast for masses, tenderness, and any discharge from the nipples.

- Palpate the areolae and the nipples for masses. Compress each nipple to determine the presence of any discharge. If a discharge is present, milk the breast along its radii to identify the discharge-producing lobe. Assess any discharge for amount, color, consistency, and odor. Note any tenderness on palpation.

The Abdomen

Inspection of the Abdomen

- Inspect the abdomen for skin integrity, contour, and symmetry.

- Observe abdominal movements associated with respiration, peristalsis, or aortic pulsations.

Auscultation of the Abdomen

- Auscultate the abdomen for bowel sounds, vascular sounds, and peritoneal friction rubs in all four quadrants. See the figure of the quadrants of the abdomen on page 133.

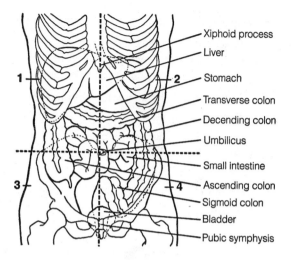

Xiphoid process
Liver
Stomach
Transverse colon
Decending colon
Umbilicus
Small intestine
Ascending colon
Sigmoid colon
Bladder
Pubic symphysis

Palpation of the Abdomen

- Perform light palpation first to detect areas of tenderness and/or muscle guarding. Systematically explore all four quadrants.

- Perform deep palpation over all four quadrants.

Palpation of the Bladder

- Palpate the area above the pubic symphysis if the client's history indicates possible urinary retention.

Musculoskeletal System

Muscles

- Inspect muscles for size. Compare the muscles on one side of the body to the corresponding muscles on the other side.

- Inspect muscles and tendons for contractures.

- Inspect the muscles for fasciculations and tremors. Inspect any tremors by having the client hold the arms out in front of the body.

- Palpate the muscles at rest to determine muscle tonicity.

- Palpate muscles while the client is active and passive for flaccidity, spasticity, and smoothness of movement.

- Test muscle strength. Compare the right side with the left side.

Bones
- Inspect the skeleton for normal structure and deformities.

- Palpate the bones to locate any areas of edema or tenderness.

Joints
- Inspect the joints for swelling.

- Palpate each joint for tenderness, smoothness of movement, swelling, crepitation, and the presence of nodules.

- Assess joint range of motion.

The Neurologic System
Gross Motor and Balance Test
There are several gross motor function and balance tests. Generally, the Romberg test and one other are conducted. The following tests may be carried out:

- Romberg test. Ask the client to stand with feet

together and arms resting at the sides, first with eyes open, then closed. Stand close during this test to prevent the client from falling.

- Walking gait
- Standing on one foot with eyes closed
- Heel-toe walking
- Toe or heel walking

Fine Motor Tests for the Upper Extremities
The following tests may be performed:

- Finger to nose
- Alternating supination and pronation of hands on knees
- Finger to nose and to the nurse's finger
- Finger to fingers
- Fingers to thumb (same hand)

Fine Motor Tests for the Lower Extremities
Ask the client to lie supine and perform these tests:

- Heel down opposite shin. Ask the client to place the heel of one foot just below the opposite knee and run the heel down the shin to the foot. Repeat with the other foot.

- Toe or ball of foot to the nurse's finger. Ask the client to touch your finger with the large toe of each foot.

Sensory Function
- Light-touch sensation. Compare the light touch sensation of symmetric areas of the body.

- Pain sensation. Assess pain sensation by asking the client to close the eyes and report whether a sharp, dull, or indistinguishable sensation is felt when you touch the skin with the sharp or dull end of a safety pin. Alternate between the sharp and dull ends, and randomly select different anatomic sites. Do not perform this test on the face, however.

Temperature Sensation
- Temperature sensation is not routinely tested if the pain sensation is found to be within normal limits.

- If pain sensation is abnormal or absent, touch the skin areas with test tubes filled with hot or cold water. Have the client report whether a hot, cold, or indistinguishable sensation is felt.

Position or Kinesthetic Sensation
- Commonly, the middle fingers and the large toes are tested for the kinesthetic sensation (sense of position).

- Ask the client to close the eyes. Move the finger or toe until it is up, down, or straight out, and ask the client to identify the position.

Tactile Discrimination
For all tests, the client's eyes must be closed. The following tests may be performed:

- One- and two-point discrimination. Alternate touching the skin with one or two pins. Ask whether the client feels one or two pinpricks.

- Stereognosis. Place familiar objects (key, paper clip, or coin) in the client's hand, and ask the client to identify them. If the client has a motor impairment of the hand, write a number or letter on the hand with a blunt instrument, and ask the client to identify it.

- Extinction phenomenon. Simultaneously stimulate two symmetric areas of the body to determine whether both points of stimulus are felt.

The Female Genitals and Inguinal Lymph Nodes

- Inspect the distribution, amount, and characteristics of pubic hair.

- Inspect the skin of the pubic area for lesions, swelling, inflammation, and presence of parasites. To assess adequately, separate the labia majora and labia minora.

- Inspect the clitoris, urethral orifice, and vaginal orifice when separating the labia minora.

- If there is inflammation or discharge at the urethral orifice, palpate Skene's glands on either side of the urethral orifice.

- Palpate Bartholin's glands.

- Assess the pelvic musculature while your gloved finger is in the vaginal orifice.

- Palpate the inguinal lymph nodes using the pads of the fingers in a rotary motion, noting any enlargement or tenderness.

The Male Genitals and Inguinal Area

- Use this as an opportunity to teach testicular self-examination (TSE).

- Inspect pubic hair distribution, amount, and characteristics.

- Inspect the penile shaft and glans for lesions, nodules, swelling, and inflammation.

- Inspect the urethral meatus for swelling, inflammation, and discharge.

- Palpate the penis for tenderness, thickening, and nodules.

- Inspect the scrotum for appearance, size, and symmetry.

- Palpate the scrotum for masses, tenderness, or lesions.

- Palpate the scrotum to assess status of the underlying testes, epididymis, and spermatic cord. Palpate the testes simultaneously for comparative purposes.

- Inspect inguinal areas for bulges while the client is standing, if possible. Have the client hold the breath and strain or bear down as though having a bowel movement.

- Palpate hernias.

The Rectum and Anus

- Inspect the anus and surrounding tissue for color, integrity, and skin lesions.

- Palpate the rectum for anal sphincter tonicity, nodules, masses, and tenderness.

- On withdrawal of the gloved finger from the rectum and anus, observe it for feces.

- For males, palpate the prostate gland through the anterior rectal wall. Note size and consistency.

- For females, palpate the cervix through the anterior rectal wall.

E. NURSING DIAGNOSES

North American Nursing Diagnosis Association (NANDA)1999-2000

Activity Intolerance
Activity Intolerance, Risk for
Adaptive Capacity, Decreased: Intracranial
Adjustment, Impaired
Adult Failure to Thrive
Airway Clearance, Ineffective
Anxiety
Anxiety, Death
Aspiration, Risk for
Autonomic Dysreflexia, Risk for
Bathing/Hygiene Self-Care Deficit
Bed Mobility, Impaired
Body Image Disturbance
Body Temperature, Risk for Altered
Breastfeeding, Effective
Breastfeeding, Ineffective
Breastfeeding, Interrupted
Breathing Pattern, Ineffective
Cardiac Output, Decreased
Caregiver Role Strain
Caregiver Role Strain, Risk for
Community Coping, Ineffective
Community Coping, Potential for Enhanced

Confusion, Acute
Confusion, Chronic
Constipation
Constipation, Colonic
Constipation, Perceived
Constipation, Risk for
Decisional Conflict (specify)
Defensive Coping
Delayed Surgical Recovery
Denial, Ineffective
Dentition, Altered
Development, Risk for Altered
Diarrhea
Disuse Syndrome, Risk for
Diversional Activity Deficit
Dressing/Grooming Self-Care Deficit
Dysreflexia
Energy Field Disturbance
Environmental Interpretation Syndrome, Impaired
Family Coping, Ineffective: Compromised
Family Coping, Ineffective: Disabling
Family Coping: Potential for Growth
Family Processes, Altered
Family Processes, Altered: Alcoholism
Fatigue
Fear
Feeding Self-Care Deficit
Fluid Volume Deficit
Fluid Volume Deficit, Risk for
Fluid Volume Excess
Fluid Volume Imbalance, Risk for
Gas Exchange, Impaired
Grieving, Anticipatory

➔

E. Nursing Diagnoses *(continued)*

Grieving, Dysfunctional
Growth and Development, Altered
Growth, Risk for Altered
Health Maintenance, Altered
Health-Seeking Behaviors (specify)
Home Maintenance Management, Impaired
Hopelessness
Hyperthermia
Hypothermia
Incontinence, Bowel
Incontinence, Functional Urinary
Incontinence, Reflex Urinary
Incontinence, Risk for Urinary Urge
Incontinence, Stress
Incontinence, Total
Incontinence, Urge
Individual Coping, Ineffective
Infant Behavior, Disorganized
Infant Behavior, Potential for Enhanced Organized
Infant Behavior, Risk for Disorganized
Infant Feeding Pattern, Ineffective
Infection, Risk for
Injury, Risk for
Knowledge Deficit (specify)
Latex Allergy Response
Latex Allergy Response, Risk for
Loneliness, Risk for
Management of Therapeutic Regimen, Effective: Individual
Management of Therapeutic Regimen, Ineffective:
    Community
Management of Therapeutic Regimen, Ineffective: Families
Management of Therapeutic Regimen, Ineffective:
    Individuals

Memory, Impaired

Nausea

Noncompliance (specify)

Nutrition, Altered: Less Than Body Requirements

Nutrition, Altered: More Than Body Requirements

Nutrition, Altered: Risk for More Than Body Requirements

Oral Mucous Membrane, Altered

Pain

Pain, Chronic

Parent/Infant/Child Attachment, Risk for Altered

Parental Role Conflict

Parenting, Altered

Parenting, Risk for Altered

Perioperative Positioning Injury, Risk for

Peripheral Neurovascular Dysfunction, Risk for

Personal Identity Disturbance

Physical Mobility, Impaired

Poisoning, Risk for

Post-Trauma Syndrome

Post-Trauma Syndrome, Risk for

Powerlessness

Protection, Altered

Rape Trauma Syndrome

Rape Trauma Syndrome: Compound Reaction

Rape Trauma Syndrome: Silent Reaction

Relocation Stress Syndrome

Role Performance, Altered

Self-Esteem Disturbance

Self-Esteem, Chronic Low

Self-Esteem, Situational Low

Self-Mutilation, Risk for

Sensory/Perceptual Alterations (specify) (Visual, Auditory, Kinesthetic, Gustatory, Tactile, Olfactory)

→

E. Nursing Diagnoses *(continued)*

Sexual Dysfunction
Sexuality Patterns, Altered
Skin Integrity, Impaired
Skin Integrity, Risk for Impaired
Sleep Deprivation
Sleep Pattern Disturbance
Social Interaction, Impaired
Social Isolation
Sorrow, Chronic
Spiritual Distress (Distress of the Human Spirit)
Spiritual Distress, Risk for
Spiritual Well-Being, Potential for Enhanced
Suffocation, Risk for
Swallowing, Impaired
Thermoregulation, Ineffective
Thought Processes, Altered
Tissue Integrity, Impaired
Tissue Perfusion, Altered (specify) (Renal, Cerebral,
    Cardiopulmonary, Gastrointestinal, Peripheral)
Toileting Self-Care Deficit
Transfer Ability, Impaired
Trauma, Risk for
Unilateral Neglect
Urinary Elimination, Altered
Urinary Retention
Ventilation, Inability to Sustain Spontaneous
Ventilatory Weaning Response, Dysfunctional
Verbal Communication, Impaired
Violence, Risk for: Self-Directed
Violence: Directed at Others, Risk for
Walking, Impaired
Wheelchair Mobility, Impaired

UNIT 3

Planning and Implementation

A. Safety Guidelines
B. Clinical Guidelines
C. Teaching and Learning Guidelines
D. Medications

A. SAFETY GUIDELINES

To be a safe practitioner, you must know your limitations, know how and when to seek information, and stay current in your field. As health care advances, techniques are modified. Attend the classes, read the literature, and make sure you are familiar with your responsibilities as set forth by your agency. For example, annual cardiopulmonary resuscitation (CPR) certification is required by most health care facilities; don't allow your certification to lapse.

Many health care agencies also have specific guidelines or procedures to follow in the event of an emergency, such as fire. Familiarize yourself with this information each time you go to a new facility. On each unit, make sure you know the location of the exit doors, the stairs, the crash cart, and fire extinguishers. The first rule of safety is preparedness.

Know your resources. Find out where on the unit the procedure manuals are kept. If you are unfamiliar with a procedure, look it up. Knowing your resources also means knowing whom you can go to with questions or to seek advice from. Your clinical instructor is one of your best safety resources. They know your level of knowledge, your clinical skill level, and your anxiety level. If you have concerns, talk them out with your instructor. Never perform skills that you are unsure of; always review the skill and seek assistance if you feel uncertain. See Chapter 31 of *Fundamentals of Nursing* for a thorough discussion of safety guidelines.

Investigate the availability of resource manuals. Does your unit have a *Physicians' Desk Reference* (PDR) or drug handbook? Be familiar with all medications that you administer: Carry a drug handbook, or consult a unit handbook before administering medications. If you still have questions, go to your instructor to talk them through. Be aware that the pharmacy staff is there to help you; pharmacists are particularly helpful for answering questions about new drugs, discussing drug-drug interactions, and planning medication schedules for clients.

Do not take unnecessary risks. Follow standard precautions to protect yourself from blood-borne pathogens. See pages 12 to 16 for a quick reference on standard precautions. To provide safe care, you must also use good body mechanics. Summaries of body mechanics guidelines and other safety guidelines are provided below.

Guidelines Related to Body Mechanics

- Start any body movement with proper alignment.

- Stand as close as possible to the object to be moved.

- Avoid stretching, reaching, and twisting, which may place the line of gravity outside your base of support.

- Before moving objects, increase your stability by widening your stance and flexing your knees, hips, and ankles.

- Adjust the working area to waist level, and keep your body close to the area.

- To prevent stretching and reaching, elevate adjustable beds and overbed tables, or lower the side rails of beds.

- When *pushing* an object, enlarge your base of support by moving your front foot forward.

- When *pulling* an object, enlarge your base of support either by moving the rear leg back (if you are facing the object) or by moving the front foot forward (if you are facing away from the object).

- Before moving objects, contract your gluteal, abdominal, leg, and arm muscles to prepare them for action.

- To move objects below your center of gravity, begin with the back and knees flexed. When lifting the weight, use your gluteal and leg muscles rather than the sacrospinal muscles of your back to exert an upward thrust.

- To prevent back strain, distribute the work load between both arms and legs.

- Always face the direction of the movement to prevent twisting of the spine and ineffective use of major muscle groups.

- When moving or carrying objects, hold them as close as possible to your center of gravity.

- To control an object's movement and keep it close to your center of gravity, pull the object toward you whenever possible rather than pushing it away.

- Provide a firm, smooth, dry bed foundation before moving a client in bed.

- Pull clients rather than push them whenever possible.

- Encourage clients to assist as much as possible by pushing or pulling themselves to reduce the muscular effort you need to expend.

- Use arms as levers whenever possible to increase lifting power.

- Use your own body weight to counteract the weight of the object you are moving. For example, lean forward when pushing an object, and rock your body weight backward when pulling an object or client toward you.

- Obtain the assistance of other persons or use mechanical devices to move objects that are too heavy for you to move alone.

- Avoid working against gravity.

- Pull, push, roll, or turn objects instead of lifting them.

- Lower the head of the client's bed before moving the client up in bed.

- Alternate rest periods with periods of muscle use to help prevent fatigue.

Preventing Falls in Hospitals

- Orient clients on admission to their surroundings, and explain the call system.

- Carefully assess the client's ability to ambulate and transfer; provide walking aids and assistance as required.

- Closely supervise the clients at risk for falls during the first few days, especially at night.

- Encourage the client to use call bell to request assistance; ensure that the bell is within reach.

- Place bedside tables and overbed tables near the bed or chair so that clients do not overreach and consequently lose their balance.

- Always keep hospital beds in the low position when not providing care so that clients can move in or out of bed easily.

- Encourage clients to use grab bars mounted in toilet and bathing areas and railings along corridors.

- Make sure nonskid bath mats are available in tubs and showers.

- Encourage the client to wear nonskid footwear.

- Keep the environment tidy, especially keep light cords from underfoot and furniture out of the way.

- Reduce poor lighting and glare, which causes clients to squint.

- Attach side rails to the beds of confused, sedated, restless, and unconscious clients, and keep the rails in place when the client is unattended.

Adult Home Hazard Appraisal

- *Walkways and stairways (inside and outside).* Note uneven sidewalks or paths, broken or loose steps, absence of hand rails or placement on only one side of stairways, insecure hand rails, congested hallways or other traffic areas, and adequacy of lighting at night.

- *Floors.* Note uneven and highly polished or slippery floors and any unanchored rugs or mats.

- *Furniture.* Note hazardous placement of furniture with sharp corners. Note chairs or stools that are too low to get into and out of or that provide inadequate support.

- *Bathroom(s).* Note the presence of grab bars around tubs and toilets, nonslip surfaces in tubs and shower stalls, adequacy of lighting for medicine cabinet, and need for raised toilet seat or bath chair in tub or shower.

- *Kitchen.* Note pilot lights (gas stove) in need of repair, inaccessible storage areas, and hazardous furniture. Check for presence of operational smoke detector.

- *Bedrooms.* Note adequacy of lighting, in particular the availability of night-lights and accessibility of light switches. Assess floors and furniture as above. Note access to bathroom.

- *Electrical.* Note unanchored and/or frayed electrical cords, overloaded outlets, and any outlets near water.

- *Fire protection.* Note the presence or absence of a fire extinguisher and fire escape plan, improper storage of combustibles (eg, gasoline) or corrosives (eg, rust remover [phosphoric acid]), and accessibility of emergency telephone numbers (fire, police).

- *Toxic substances.* Note appropriate storage of medicines or toxic substances such as cleaning solutions. Note medications kept beyond date of expiration and improperly labeled cleaning solutions.

Steps to Follow in the Event of Fire

- Activate the fire alarm if one is nearby.

- Notify the hospital switchboard of the location of the fire.

- Evacuate clients who are in immediate danger. First, direct ambulatory clients to a safe area, or enlist their help in moving clients in wheelchairs. This clears the area for the evacuation of nonambulatory clients, who can be moved in a stretcher or bed, carried, or dragged on sheets and blankets.

- If the fire is small, use the fire extinguisher.

- Close windows and doors in the area of the fire to reduce ventilation.

- Turn off oxygen and any electrical appliances in the vicinity.

- Clear fire exits, if necessary.

- Contain smoke as necessary by placing damp cloths or blankets around the outside edges of doors.

- Protect clients from smoke inhalation by giving them wet washcloths through which to breathe.

Discharge Planning and Home Care Assessment

Client/Environment

- Self-care abilities for hygiene and toileting
- Self-care abilities for medication administration
- Self-care abilities for wound care
- Facilities: presence of running water, garbage, bathroom to facilitate wound care and contain potentially infectious materials

Family

- Caregiver availability, skills, and willingness
- Family concerns about caregiving

Community

- Resources

B. CLINICAL GUIDELINES

Fluid and Electrolyte Balance
Assess to Determine

- The usual amount and type of fluids ingested each day.

- Foods rich in protein, sodium, potassium, and calcium eaten each day.

- Any recent changes in food or fluid intake and reason (eg, presence of nausea, pain, anorexia, or dysphagia).

- Any recent changes in frequency or amount of urine output.

- Major losses of body fluid through vomiting, diarrhea, excessive perspiration, or other route (eg, drainage from gastrointestinal function, ileostomy, colostomy, or burn sites).

- History of any long-term or recent disease processes that might disrupt fluid, electrolyte, and acid-base balance: kidney disease, heart disease, high blood pressure, diabetes mellitus, diabetes insipidus, thyroid or parathyroid disorders, asthma, emphysema, severe trauma, or other chronic disease states (eg, cancer, colitis, ileitis).

- Medication therapy that could affect fluid and electrolyte balance: diuretics, steroids, potassium supplements, or aldosterone inhibitor agents.

- Recent treatments that could affect fluid and electrolyte balance, such as dialysis; total parenteral nutrition; tube drainage (eg, nasogastric or intestinal suction); or tube feedings.

Assess the Client for
- Signs that indicate insufficient hydration: excessive thirst, dry skin and mucous membranes, concentrated urine, reduced urine output, poor tissue turgor, depressed periorbital spaces.

- Signs indicating excessive hydration: swollen ankles, difficulty breathing, sudden weight gain, ascites, moist crackles (rales) in lungs.

- Signs that might indicate an electrolyte or acid-base imbalance: loss of mental alertness; disorientation; faintness; muscle weakness, twitching, cramps, fatigue, pain, or spasm; abnormal sensations (eg, burning, prickling, tingling); abdominal cramps or distention; heart palpitations.

Obtain Clinical Measurements
- Baseline and daily weight. Rapid losses or gains of 5% or more of total body weight indicate moderate to severe fluid volume deficit or excess.

- Vital signs. *Body temperature:* An increased body temperature may indicate hypernatremic dehydration; a decreased body temperature may result from hypovolemia. *Pulse rate:* An increased pulse rate and a weak, thready pulse may occur with fluid volume deficit or potassium excess. *Respiration:* An increased rate and depth of respiration may cause carbonic acid deficit (respiratory alkalosis); shallow respirations may create a carbonic acid excess (respiratory acidosis). Either may be a compensatory mechanism for metabolic acid-base imbalances. *Blood pressure:* An elevated systolic blood pressure may indicate a fluid volume excess; a sudden decreased systolic pressure exceeding 10 mm Hg usually indicates a fluid volume deficit.

- 24-hour fluid intake and output.

Review Results of Laboratory Tests
- Serum electrolyte levels
- Hematocrit
- Urine pH
- Urine specific gravity
- Arterial blood gases (ABGs)

Identify Clients at Risk for Fluid and Electrolyte Imbalances
- Postoperative clients
- Clients with severe trauma or burns
- Clients with chronic diseases, such as congestive heart failure, diabetes, chronic obstructive lung disease, and cancer
- Clients who are permitted nothing by mouth (NPO)
- Clients with intravenous infusions

- Clients with retention catheters and urinary drainage systems

- Clients with special drainages or suctions, such as a nasogastric suction

- Clients receiving diuretics

- Clients experiencing excessive fluid losses and requiring increased intake

- Clients who retain fluids

- Clients with fluid restrictions

- Elderly clients who may not be taking in the fluids they need

- Clients unable to respond to the thirst sensation, (eg, comatose clients)

- Clients receiving electrolyte therapy (eg, potassium supplements)

- Clients unable to communicate desire for fluid (eg, very young clients)

- Clients with very high or very low total body water

Key Elements: Monitoring Fluid Intake and Output

- To assess fluid balance, determine the client's intake and output (I & O), and observe the client for signs of dehydration or overhydration.

- Monitor I & O for all clients (a) whose oral fluid intake is insufficient, (b) who are experiencing excessive fluid loss via normal or abnormal routes, (c) who are retaining fluid, or (d) who are taking medications that alter fluid output.

- Weigh daily clients who are retaining fluid or receiving diuretics.

Key Elements: Facilitating Normal or Increased Fluid Intake

- Explain to the client the reason for the required intake and the specific amount needed. This gives the client a rationale for the requirement and thus promotes compliance.

- Establish a 24-hour plan for ingesting the fluids. Generally, half of the total volume is ingested during the day shift, and the other half is divided between the evening and night shifts, with the majority ingested during the evening shift. For example, if 2500 mL is to be ingested in 24 hours, the plan may specify that 1500 mL be ingested in the 7–3 shift, 700 mL in the 3–11 shift, and 300 mL in the 11–7 shift. To prevent the need to urinate during sleeping hours, clients should avoid ingesting large amounts of fluid before bedtime.

- Set short-term outcomes that the client can realistically meet. For example, the client might ingest a glass of fluid every hour while awake or a pitcher of water by 12 noon.

- Identify fluids the client likes, and make available a variety of those items. Examples may include fruit juices, tea, coffee, and milk (if allowed).

- Help clients to select foods that tend to become liquid at room temperature (eg, gelatin, ice cream, sherbert, custard), if these are allowed.

- For clients who are confined to bed, supply appropriate cups, glasses, and straws to facilitate appropriate fluid intake. Keep the fluids within easy reach.

- Make sure fluids are served at the appropriate temperature: hot fluids hot, and cold fluids iced and cold.

- Encourage clients to participate in maintaining the fluid intake record, when possible. This helps them determine whether they are achieving preestablished goals.

- Be alert for the cultural implications of food and fluids. Some cultures may restrict certain foods and fluids and view others as having healing properties.

Key Elements: Helping Clients Restrict Fluid Intake

- Explain the reason for the restricted intake. Be sure also to explain how much and what types of fluids are permitted orally. Many clients need to be informed that ice chips, gelatin, and ice cream, for example, are considered fluid.

- Help the client decide how to allocate the total amount of fluid allowed: how much to take with each meal, between meals, before bedtime, and with medications. Generally, half of the total volume is scheduled during the day shift, when the client is most active, receives two meals, and, often, most oral medications. A large part of the remainder is scheduled for the evening shift to permit the client to take fluids with meals and during evening visits.

- Identify fluids the client likes, and make sure that these are provided, unless contraindicated. A client who is allowed only 200 mL of fluid for breakfast, for example, should receive the type of fluid the client favors.

- Set short-term goals that make the fluid restriction more tolerable. For example, schedule a specified amount of fluid at 1- or 2-hour intervals between meals. Some clients may prefer fluids between meals only, because the food provided at mealtime may help relieve feelings of thirst.

- Provide the client with small fluid containers that make the container appear to contain more fluid than it actually does.

- Periodically offer the client ice chips as an alternative to water. Ice chips occupy twice the volume of an equal amount of water.

- Help clients rinse their mouths with water if they can do so without swallowing the fluid.

- Ensure meticulous oral care.

- Instruct the client to avoid ingesting or chewing salty or sweet foods (hard candy or gum), because these foods tend to produce thirst. Sugarless gum may be an alternative for some clients.

- Encourage the client to participate in maintaining the fluid intake record, when possible.

CLINICAL GUIDELINES

Individualizing Care for Clients with Pain

- Establish a trusting relationship. Convey your concern and acknowledge that you believe the client is experiencing pain. A trusting relationship encourages the client to express thoughts and feelings and enhances the effectiveness of planned pain therapies.

- Assess the source of the pain carefully. The source of the pain may not always be what is apparent. For example, the post-operative client who has had abdominal surgery may complain of pain related to a headache or other discomfort.

- Consider the client's ability and willingness to participate actively in pain-relief measures. Excessively fatigued or sedated clients or those who have altered levels of consciousness are less able to actively participate.

- Use a variety of pain-relief measures. It is thought that using more than one measure has an additive effect in relieving pain. Two measures that should always be part of a pain relief plan are (a) establishing a trusting client-nurse relationship and (b) client teaching. Because a client's pain may vary throughout a 24-hour period, different types of pain relief are often indicated during that time.

- Provide measures to relieve pain before it becomes severe. For example, it is better to provide an analgesic before pain is expected than to wait for the client to complain of pain, when a larger dose may be required.

- Use pain-relief measures that the client believes are effective. It has been recognized that clients are often knowledgeable about measures that are effective in relieving their own pain. Therefore, incorporate the client's measures into a pain relief plan, unless they are harmful.

- Consider the client's willingness to participate actively in pain-relief measures.

- Base the choice of the pain-relief measure on the client's report of the severity of the pain. If a client reports mild pain, an analgesic such as aspirin may be indicated, whereas a client who reports severe pain may require a more potent relief measure.

- If a pain-relief measure proves to be ineffective, encourage the client to try it once or twice more before abandoning it. Anxiety may inhibit the effectiveness of a pain-relief measure, and some approaches, such as distraction strategies, require practice before they become effective.

- Maintain an unbiased attitude (open mind) about what may relieve the pain. New ways to relieve pain are continually being developed. It is not always possible to explain why a pain-relief measure works; however, you should support a measure unless it is harmful.

- Keep trying. Do *not* ignore a client because pain persists in spite of taking measures to relieve it. In these circumstances, reassess the pain, and consider other pain-relief measures.

- Prevent harm to the client. Pain therapy should not increase discomfort or harm the client.

- Educate the client and support persons about pain. Inform them about possible causes, precipitating and alleviating factors, and alternatives to drug therapy. Correct any misconceptions.

Key Elements: Pain-Distraction Techniques

- *Slow, rhythmic breathing.* Instruct the client to stare at an object, inhale slowly through the nose while counting from 1 to 4, and then exhale slowly through the mouth while counting to 4 again. Encourage the client to concentrate on the sensation of breathing and to picture a restful scene. Continue until a rhythmic pattern is established.

- *Massage and slow, rhythmic breathing.* Instruct the client to breathe rhythmically while massaging a painful body part with stroking or circular movements.

- *Rhythmic singing and tapping.* Ask the client to select a well-liked song and focus attention on its words and rhythm. Encourage the client to mouth or sing the words and tap a finger or foot. Loud, fast songs are best for intense pain.

- *Active listening.* Have the client listen to music and concentrate on the rhythm by tapping a finger or foot.

- *Guided imagery*. Ask the client to close the eyes and imagine and describe something pleasurable. As the client describes the image, ask about the sights, sounds, and smells imagined, encouraging the client to provide details.

CLINICAL GUIDELINES

Respiratory Function
Assess to Determine

- *Current respiratory problems.* What recent changes has the client experienced in breathing pattern (eg, shortness of breath, difficulty breathing, need to be in upright position to breathe, or rapid and shallow breathing)?

- *History of respiratory disease.* Has the client had colds, allergies, croup, asthma, tuberculosis, bronchitis, pneumonia, or emphysema? How frequently have these occurred? How long did they last? And how were they treated?

- *The presence of a cough.* Is it productive or non-productive? If the cough is productive, when is sputum produced? What is the amount, color, thickness, odor, and character of the sputum (eg, thick, frothy, pink, rusty, or blood-tinged)?

- *Lifestyle.* Does the client smoke? If so, how much? Does any member of the client's family smoke? Are there any occupational hazards (eg, noxious fumes)?

- *Pain.* Does the client experience any pain associated with breathing or activity? Where is the pain located? What words does the client use to describe the pain? How long does it last, and how does it affect breathing? What activities precede the pain?

- *Medication history.* Has the client taken or does the client take any over-the-counter or prescription medications for breathing? Which ones? And what are the dosages, times taken, and effects on the client, including side effects?

Observe the Client's
- Breathing pattern (rate, rhythm, depth, and quality). Note any signs of hyperventilation or hypoventilation, tachypnea, or bradypnea.

- Ease or effort of breathing and posture assumed for breathing (eg, orthopneic).

- Breath sounds audible without amplification (eg, stridor, stertor, wheeze, bubbling).

- Chest movements (eg, retractions, flail chest, or paradoxical breathing). Note the specific location of retractions: intercostal, substernal, suprasternal, or supraclavicular. Note also the presence of tracheal tug.

- Clinical signs of hypoxia or anoxia, such as increased pulse rate, rapid or deep respirations, cyanosis of the skin and nail beds, restlessness, anxiety, dizziness (vertigo), or faintness (syncope).

- The location of any surgical incision in relation to the muscles needed for breathing. An incision can impede appropriate lung expansion.

Palpate for
- Respiratory excursion.

- Lungs for vocal (tactile) fremitus.

Percuss the Chest for
- Diaphragmatic excursion.
- Chest sounds (flatness, dullness, resonance, hyperresonance, tympany).

Auscultate the Lungs for
- Breath sounds (normal, adventitious, or absent).

Determine the Results of
- Sputum analysis.
- Venous blood samples (eg, complete blood count).
- Arterial blood samples (blood gases).
- Pulmonary function tests.
- Pulse oximetry.

Abnormal Breathing Patterns and Breath Sounds
Breathing Patterns
Rate
- Tachypnea—rapid respiration marked by quick, shallow breaths.
- Bradypnea—abnormally slow breathing.
- Apnea—cessation of breathing.

Volume/Depth
- Hyperventilation—an increase in the amount of air in the lungs; characterized by prolonged and deep breaths; may be associated with anxiety.

- Hypoventilation—reduction in the amount of air in the lungs; characterized by shallow respirations.

Rhythm
- Cheyne-Stokes respirations—rhythmic waxing and waning of respirations, from very deep to very shallow breathing and temporary apnea; often associated with cardiac failure, increased intracranial pressure, or brain damage.

Ease or Effort
- Dyspnea—difficult and labored breathing during which the individual has a persistent, unsatisfied need for air and feels distressed.

- Orthopnea—ability to breathe only in upright sitting or standing positions.

Breath Sounds
Audible Without Amplification
- Stridor—a shrill, harsh sound heard during inspiration; due to laryngeal obstruction.

- Stertor—snoring or sonorous respiration, usually due to a partial obstruction of the upper airway.

- Wheeze—continuous, high-pitched musical squeak or whistling sound occurring on expiration and sometimes on inspiration when air moves through a narrowed or partially obstructed airway.

- Bubbling—gurgling sounds heard as air passes through moist secretions in the respiratory tract.

Audible by Stethoscope
- Crackles (also called *rales*)—dry or wet crackling sounds similar to the sound produced by rolling

a lock of hair near the ear; generally heard on inspiration as air moves through accumulated moist secretions. *Fine to medium crackles* occur when air passes through moisture in small air passages and alveoli; *medium to coarse crackles* occur when air passes through moisture in the brochioles, bronchi, and trachea.

- Gurgles (also called *rhonchi*)—coarse, leathery, or grating sound produced by the rubbing together of inflamed pleural tissues.

Chest Movements

- Intercostal retraction—indrawing between the ribs.

- Substernal retraction—indrawing beneath the breastbone.

- Suprasternal retraction—indrawing above the breastbone.

- Supraclavicular retraction—indrawing above the clavicles.

- Tracheal tug—indrawing and downward pull of the trachea during inspiration.

- Flail chest—the ballooning out of the chest wall through injured rib spaces; results in paradoxical breathing, during which the chest wall balloons on expiration but is depressed or sucked inward on inspiration.

Secretions and Coughing

- Hemoptysis—the presence of blood in the sputum.

- Productive cough—a cough accompanied by expectorated secretions.

- Nonproductive cough—a dry, harsh cough without secretions.

Key Elements: Oropharyngeal and Nasopharyngeal Suctioning

- Assess the client's respirations (rate, depth, rhythm, character, and sound); skin and mucous membrane color; difficulty breathing; lung sounds (by auscultation); ability to cough and produce sputum; and level of consciousness before and after suctioning.

- Maintain sterility of the suction catheter, flushing solution, and gauzes used to wipe the catheter.

- Position conscious clients appropriately:

  a. For nasal suctioning, hyperextend the neck.

  b. For oral suctioning, turn the head to one side.

  c. For tracheal suctioning, hyperextend the head and have the client extend the tongue.

  d. For the left bronchus, turn the head to the right.

  e. For the right bronchus, turn the head to the left.

- In the unconscious client, prevent aspiration of sputum by positioning the person in the lateral position.

- Before the procedure, measure the correct length for catheter insertion.

- Moisten the catheter tip before insertion.

- Insert the catheter *without applying suction*. For tracheal suctioning, insert the catheter while the client inhales.

- Never force the catheter against an obstruction.

- Gently rotate the catheter while applying suction.

- Prevent or minimize hypoxia: Apply suction for no more than 15 seconds each time and for no longer than 5 minutes in total.

- Encourage deep breathing and coughing between suctions.

- For the client on a ventilator, hyperventilate the client prior to suctioning.

- Flush the catheter between suctions.

- Change suction collection bottles and tubing at least daily.

CLINICAL GUIDELINES

Tube Feedings
Assess to Determine

- Allergies to any food in the feeding. Common ingredients in feedings include milk, sugar, water, eggs, and vegetable oil.

- Bowel sounds prior to each feeding (or every 4 to 8 hours for continuous feedings) to determine intestinal activity.

- Abdominal distention at least daily. Measure the client's abdominal girth at the umbilicus. A distended abdomen may indicate intolerance to a previous feeding.

- Correct placement of the tube before feedings.

- Presence of regurgitation and feelings of fullness after feedings.

- Dumping syndrome. Jejunostomy clients may experience nausea, vomiting, diarrhea, cramps, pallor, sweating, heart palpitations, increased pulse rate, and fainting after a feeding. These are signs of dumping syndrome, which results when hypertonic foods and liquids suddenly distend the jejunum. To make the intestinal contents isotonic, body fluids shift rapidly from the client's vascular system. Smaller, more frequent feedings, slower feedings, and a longer adjustment period may relieve dumping.

- Presence of diarrhea, constipation, or flatulence. The lack of bulk in liquid feedings may cause constipation. The presence of concentrated ingredients may cause diarrhea and flatulence.

- Urine for sugar and acetone. Monitor the client's urine every 4 to 6 hours for the first 48 hours after initial feedings are begun.

- Hydration status. Measure the client's fluid intake and output, and note complaints of thirst. Additional water may need to be instilled between feedings.

Before Administering the Feeding
- Check the expiration date of the feeding.

- Warm the feeding to room temperature.

- Confirm correct placement of the tube.

- Aspirate residual stomach contents, measure the amount, and check with the nurse in charge to determine whether to reinstill the contents or to continue the feeding.

- Remove air from the feeding tubes of the feeding bag and prefilled bottles with drip chambers.

- Deliver the feeding over the desired length of time.

After the Feeding
- Rinse the nasogastric tube with water.

- Clamp the nasogastric tube before all of the rinse solution has run through.

- Have the client remain in Fowler's position or a slightly elevated right lateral position for at least 30 minutes.

Key Elements:
Inserting a Nasogastric Tube

- Minimize discomfort by positioning the client appropriately, lubricating the tube, and working cooperatively with the client.

- Never force the tube against resistance.

- Confirm correct placement of the tube.

- Secure the tube appropriately to the client's nose or nose and cheek.

Key Elements: Administering a Nasogastric or Orogastric Feeding
Before Administering the Feeding

- Assess the client for feelings of abdominal distention, belching, loose stools, flatus, or pain; assess the client for bowel sounds and allergies to foods in the feeding.

- Check the expiration date of the feeding.

- Warm the feeding to room temperature.

- Confirm correct placement of the tube.

- Aspirate residual stomach contents, measure the amount, and check with the nurse in charge to determine whether to reinstill the contents or to continue the feeding.

- Remove air from the feeding tubes of the burette and prefilled bottles with drip chambers.

- Deliver the feeding over the desired length of time.

During the Feeding
- Hold and cuddle an infant, and provide a pacifier.

After the Feeding
- Rinse the nasogastric tube with water.

- Clamp the nasogastric tube before all of the rinse solution has run through.

- Have the client remain in Fowler's position or a slightly elevated right lateral position for at least 30 minutes.

Key Elements: Removing a Nasogastric Tube
- Turn off the suction, and disconnect the tube from suction.

- Clamp the tubing before removal.

- Don disposable gloves.

- Withdraw the tubing while the client holds the breath.

Key Elements: Administering a Gastrostomy or Jejunostomy Feeding
Before the Feeding
- Confirm whether the feeding is to be withheld if more than 50 mL of stomach or jejunal contents are aspirated.

- Position the client appropriately.
- Lubricate tubes before inserting them into stomas.
- Aspirate, measure, and reinstill (if indicated) stomach or jejunal contents.

After the Feeding
- Rinse the tube with water.
- Position the client appropriately for at least 30 minutes.
- Clean the peristomal, skin, and inspect it for irritation.
- Apply peristomal skin protectants and appropriate dressings.

CLINICAL GUIDELINES

Urinary Elimination
Assess to Determine
- Client's usual patterns and frequency of urination. Ask at what approximate times voiding occurs each day.

Note Recent Alterations in Voiding
- Passage of large amounts of urine.

- Passage of small amounts of urine.

- Voiding at more frequent intervals.

- Trouble getting to the bathroom in time or feeling of urgency to void.

- Painful voiding.

- Difficulty starting urine stream.

- Frequent dribbling of urine or feeling of bladder fullness associated with voiding small amounts of urine.

- Reduced force of stream.

- Accidental leakage of urine. If so, when this occurs (eg, when coughing, laughing, or sneezing; at night; during the day).

Obtain the Medical History
of Urinary Elimination Problems

- Urinary tract infections of the kidney, bladder, or urethra.

- Urinary calculi.

- Urinary tract surgery, such as kidney surgery, bladder surgery, prostate removal, or other surgical procedures that alter urinary routes (eg, ureterostomy).

- Cardiovascular disease, such as hypertension or heart disease.

- Chronic diseases that alter urinary characteristics or impair urinary function, such as diabetes mellitus, neurologic disease (eg, multiple sclerosis), and cancer.

Assess the Volume and Characteristics
of the Client's Urine

- Time when the client last voided and the amount. Volumes of less than 30 mL or more than 500 mL per hour must be reported immediately.

- Dark, cloudy, or discolored urine.

- Presence of mucus plugs.

- Offensive odor.

Determine Factors Influencing
Urinary Elimination

- *Medications.* Any medications that could increase urinary output (eg, diuretics) or cause retention of urine (eg, anticholinergic-antispasmodic drugs, antidepressant-antipsychotic drugs, antiparkinsonism drugs, antihistamines, antihypertensives) or that may discolor urine (eg, Azo Gantrisin, multivitamins, amitripine hydrochloride [Elavil]). Note specific medication and dosage.

- *Fluid intake.* Amount and kind of fluid taken each day (eg, 6 glasses of water, 5 cups of coffee, 3 cola drinks with or without caffeine).

- *Environmental factors.* Any problems with toileting (mobility, dexterity with clothing, toilet seat too low, facility without grab bar).

- *Presence of long-term catheter.* How the client cares for the catheter, any discomfort with it or other problems, and how the nurse can help manage it.

- *Disease.* Any illnesses other than urinary tract disease that may affect urinary function, such as hypertension, heart disease, neurologic disease (eg, multiple sclerosis), cancer, prostatic enlargement, diabetes mellitus, or diabetes insipidus.

- *Diagnostic procedures.* Recent procedures, such as cystoscopy or spinal anesthetic.

Determine the Presence of Pain
- *Bladder pain.* Pain over the suprapubic region.

- *Kidney or flank pain.* Pain between ribs and ileum, which may spread to the abdomen and be associated with nausea and vomiting.

  or

  Pain at the costovertebral angle, which may radiate to the umbilicus.

- *Ureteral pain.* Pain in the back, which may radiate to abdomen, upper thigh, testes, or labia.

Review Data from Diagnostic Tests and Examinations

- pH under 4.5 or over 8.
- Specific gravity under 1.010 or over 1.025.
- Presence of glucose or acetone.
- Presence of occult or visible blood.
- Presence of protein, urobilinogen, or nitrite.
- Presence of microorganisms.
- Presence of obstructions.
- Blood serum: blood urea nitrogen (BUN), creatinine, sodium, potassium.

Key Elements: Female Urinary Catheterization Using a Straight Catheter

- Determine whether the amount of urine drained is to be limited.
- Obtain assistance for a client who needs help to maintain the required position.
- Clean the perineal area before catheterization.
- Use strict aseptic technique.
- Lubricate the insertion tip of the catheter before swabbing the labia with antiseptic.
- Keep the labia apart once the meatus is cleaned.
- Pick up and insert the catheter with your uncontaminated, sterile, gloved hand.

- Do not force a catheter beyond a major resistance.

- Assess the amount, color, and clarity of the urine.

Key Elements: Male Urinary Catheterization Using a Straight Catheter

- See also key elements of female urinary catheterization.

- Position the client appropriately to relax the abdominal and perineal muscles.

- Retract the foreskin of an uncircumcised client, and keep it back during the catheterization.

- Lift the penis perpendicular to the body before catheterization.

Key Elements: Inserting a Retention Catheter

- See also key elements of using a straight catheter. See the accompanying illustrations on page 182.

- Test the balloon before insertion to see that it is intact.

- Before inflating the balloon of the catheter, insert the catheter an additional 2.5 to 5 cm (1 to 2 in) beyond the point at which urine began to flow.

- Inflate the balloon with no more fluid than the balloon size indicates.

- After balloon inflation, apply slight tension on

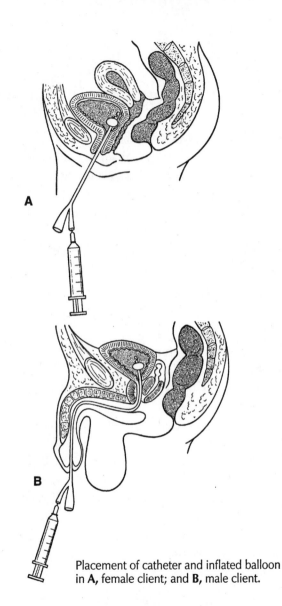

Placement of catheter and inflated balloon in **A,** female client; and **B,** male client.

the catheter to check that the balloon is well anchored in the bladder, then move the catheter slightly back into the bladder.

- Tape the catheter to the client appropriately.

- Make sure the drainage system allows free flow of urine and is well sealed or closed.

Key Elements: Removing a Retention Catheter

- Wear gloves.

- Deflate the balloon completely before removing it from the urethra.

- Observe the intactness of the catheter.

- Measure the urine in the drainage bag.

- Assess the frequency and amount of urine voided after catheter removal.

CLINICAL GUIDELINES

Fecal Elimination
Assess to Determine

- *Defecation pattern.* What is the frequency and time of day of the client's defecation? Has this pattern changed recently? Does it ever change? If so, does the client know what factors affect it?

- *Behavioral patterns.* The client's use of laxatives, fluids, and exercise to maintain the normal defecation pattern? What routines does the client follow to maintain the usual defecation pattern (eg, a glass of hot lemon juice with breakfast or a long walk before breakfast)?

- *Diet.* What foods does the client believe affect defecation? What foods does the client typically eat? What food does the client always avoid? Does the client take meals at a regular time?

- *Fluid intake.* What amount and kind of fluid does the client take each day (eg, 6 glasses of water, 5 cups of coffee)?

- *Exercise.* What is the client's usual daily exercise pattern? Obtain specific details; avoid asking whether the client's exercise is sufficient, because people's ideas of what is sufficient differ.

- *Use of elimination aids.* What routines does the client follow to maintain usual defecation pattern? Does the client use natural aids (eg, specific foods or fluids), laxatives, or enemas to maintain elimination?

- *Medications.* Has the client taken any medications that could affect the gastrointestinal tract (eg, iron in multivitamin supplements, antihistamines in cold preparations, antacids, narcotic analgesics)?

- *Pertinent illness or surgery.* Has the client had any surgery or illness that affects the intestinal tract? Are any ostomies (eg, a colostomy or ileostomy) present?

Assess the Client's

- *Vital signs: (pulse, respirations, and blood pressure)* for baseline data, particularly before administering commercial enemas or digitally removing a fecal impaction.

- *Abdominal distention.* Distention will appear as an overall outward protuberance of the abdomen, with the skin appearing tight and tense. When palpated, the abdomen feels firm. Measure a distended abdomen at the level of the umbilicus by placing a tape measure around the body. Repeated measurements will indicate whether the distention is increasing or decreasing.

- *Bowel sounds.* Auscultate all four abdominal quadrants for 5 to 15 seconds to determine the degree of activity or frequency of sounds.

- *Consistency and color of feces.* Normal feces are brown and formed but soft and moist. Note color of feces. For example, black, tarry feces may indicate the presence of blood from the stomach or small intestine; acholic feces usually indicate the absence of bile; and green or orange stools may indicate the presence of an intestinal infection. Food may also affect the color of feces; for example, beets can color stool red or sometimes green. Medications, too, can alter the color of feces; iron, for example, can make stool black.

- *Presence of constipation, diarrhea, or fecal incontinence.*

- *Perianal region and anus.* Inspect these areas for discolorations, inflammations, scars, lesions, fissures, fistulas, or hemorrhoids. Note the color, size, location, and consistency of any lesion.

- *Presence of abdominal or rectal pain.*

- *Presence of flatulence and signs associated with flatulence,* such as eructations and their frequency and the passage of flatus by the rectum. Also assess respiratory rate. Flatulence can cause pressure on the diaphragm, resulting in difficult respirations.

Identify Clients at Risk for Developing Fecal Elimination Problems
- Clients who have insufficient fluid or roughage in the diet.

- Clients who do not exercise sufficiently.

- Individuals who use constipating medications.

- Persons who ingest excessive gas-forming foods.

Key Elements: Administering an Enema

For All Enemas

- Determine the type and purpose of the enema and whether a physician's order is required.

- Position the client appropriately.

- Wear gloves.

- Assess the returns.

Cleansing Enema

- Use the correct type, amount, and temperature of solution.

- To remove air, flush the tubing before administering the enema.

- Lubricate the rectal tube before insertion.

- Direct the insertion tube toward the client's umbilicus.

- Ask the client to take a deep breath during tube insertion.

- Hold the solution container at the correct height.

- Administer the solution slowly, and start and stop the flow of solution temporarily when indicated.

Commercial Enema

- Follow the manufacturer's instructions.

Retention Enema

- Instruct client to retain the enema at least 30 minutes.

CLINICAL GUIDELINES

Pressure Areas
Assess to Determine

- The client's need for supportive devices, such as pillows, rolled or folded towels, foam rubber supports, footboard, hand rolls, wrist splints, or sandbags by assessing the client's:

  a. *Adipose tissue.* A client who has ample adipose tissue generally requires less support and cushioning than the emaciated person while in a back-lying position, but greater support to maintain a lateral position.

  b. *Skeletal structure.* Both the amount and the type of support needed vary according to the individual's skeletal structure. A person with a marked lumbar lordosis requires more lumbar support than one with a slight lumbar curvature.

  c. *Health status.* A person who has flaccid or spastic paralysis requires supportive devices. The support differs with the client's specific health status.

  d. *Discomfort.* A person who experiences pain during movement requires more support during movement than one who can move without pain. A person who is unconscious is unable to indicate discomfort and will need appropriate support and change of position at least every two hours.

e. *Skin condition.* People who have nutrition problems and/or impaired circulation require more cushioning of the pressure points to prevent skin breakdown than do healthy people.

f. *Ability to move.* People who can move in bed can change position frequently. The client who is unable to move (eg, the unconscious client) requires support so that muscles do not become strained.

g. *Hydration.* Dehydrated clients are at greater risk of pressure-sore formation than well-hydrated clients and therefore need more support under pressure areas.

Assess the Client's

- Strength and ability to move before the change of position, and obtain assistance as required. Appropriate assistance reduces the risk of muscle strain and body injury, to both the client and nurse.

- Pressure areas of the body for any whitish or reddened spots. This discoloration, which can be caused by impaired blood circulation to the area, should disappear in a few minutes when rubbing restores circulation. See the illustrations on page 190 for the location of pressure areas.

- Pressure areas of the body for abrasions and excoriations. An abrasion (wearing away of the skin) can occur when skin rubs against a sheet, such as

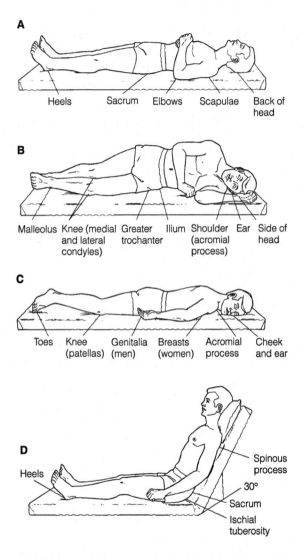

Body pressure areas in **A**, supine position; **B**, lateral position; **C**, prone position; **D**, Fowler's position.

when the client is pulled. Excoriations (loss of superficial layers of the skin) can occur when the skin has prolonged contact with body secretions or excretions, or with dampness in skinfolds.

- Stage of pressure sores, if present. The four stages of pressure sores are described as follows (USDHHS, 1992, p. 8):

  Stage I: Nonblanchable erythema of intact skin

  Stage II: Partial-thickness skin loss involving the epidermis and/or dermis

  Stage III: Full-thickness skin loss involving damage or necrosis of subcutaneous tissue that may extend down to, but not through, underlying fascia

  Stage IV: Full-thickness skin loss involving extensive destruction or damage to muscle, bone, and supporting structures

Palpate (with warm hands)

- The surface temperature of the skin over the pressure areas. Normally, the temperature is the same as that of the surrounding skin. Increased temperature is abnormal and may be due to inflammation or blood trapped in the area. A decreased temperature indicates impaired circulation.

- Over bony prominences and dependent body areas for the presence of edema. Edema will feel spongy on palpation.

Key Elements: Treating Pressure Sores

- Minimize direct pressure on the sore. Reposition the client at least every 2 hours. Make a schedule, and record position changes on the client's chart.

- Clean the pressure sore daily. Use a method consistent with the stage of the ulcer and agency protocol.

- Clean and dress the sore using surgical asepsis. Refrain from using antiseptics, such as alcohol, that are vasoconstrictors and reduce blood flow to the area.

- If the pressure sore is infected, obtain a sample of the drainage for culture and sensitivity to antiseptic agents.

- Reduce friction by applying a small amount of cornstarch to the bedsheet.

- Reduce shearing force by keeping the head of the bed flat or elevated to a maximum of 30 degrees, unless contraindicated by the client's condition.

- If the client cannot keep weight off the pressure sore, use pressure-relieving devices, such as an egg crate mattress.

- Teach the client to move, if only slightly, to relieve pressure.

- Encourage ambulation or sitting in a wheelchair as the client's condition permits.

- Provide range-of-motion (ROM) exercises as the client's condition permits.

Dressings for Pressure Ulcers

Dressing	Mechanism of Action	STAGE I	II	III	IV
Dry gauze	Wicks drainage away from wound surface	No	No	Yes	Yes
Moist gauze	Maintains a moist wound environment while wicking drainage away from surface	No	No	?	?
Moist-to-dry gauze	Debrides necrotic and healthy tissue nonselectively	No	No	?	?
Transparent adhesive	Traps serous exudate and provides a moist wound	Yes	Yes	No	No
Hydrocolloid	Reacts with wound fluid to create a soft gel that promotes granulation and epithelialization	Yes	Yes	?	No
Polyurethane foam	Absorbs exudate and maintains a moist wound	No	Yes	?	No
Absorptive dressing	Absorbs exudate and debris while maintaining a moist environment	No	No	Yes	?
Hydrogel	Maintains a moist environment	No	Yes	Yes	No

Source: J. Maklebust and M. Sieggreen, *Pressure ulcers: Guidelines for prevention and nursing management* (West Dundee, IL: S-N Publications, 1991), as cited in J. Maklebust, Pressure ulcer update. *RN*, December 1991, 54, 61. Used with permission.

CLINICAL GUIDELINES

Healing Wounds
Assess to Determine
Appearance
- Inspect color of wound and surrounding area and approximation of wound edges.

Size
- Note size and location of dehiscence, if present. For wounds healing by secondary intention, measure the length, width, and depth in centimeters.

Drainage
- Observe location, color, consistency, odor, and degree of saturation of dressings. Note number of gauzes saturated or diameter of drainage on gauze.

Swelling
- Wearing sterile gloves, palpate wound edges for tension and tautness of tissues; minimal to moderate swelling is normal in early stages of wound healing.

Pain
- Expect severe to moderate postoperative pain for 3 to 5 days; persistent severe pain or sudden

onset of severe pain may indicate internal hemorrhaging or infection.

Drains or Tubes

- Inspect drain security and placement, amount and character of drainage, and functioning of collecting apparatus, if present.

Key Elements: Changing a Dry Sterile Dressing

- Support the adjacent skin when removing adhesive tape.

- Pull tape toward the wound rather than away from it.

- Wear disposable gloves when removing moist outer dressings.

- Use sterile forceps or gloves to remove under dressings.

- Support a drain appropriately when removing dressings.

- Use separate sterile forceps to clean and dress the wound.

- Use a separate swab for each cleaning stroke.

- Clean the wound from the least contaminated to the most contaminated area.

- Clean a drain site after the incision.

- Dry the wound appropriately.

- Assess the wound appearance and drainage accurately.

- Apply sufficient dressings to cover the wound and absorb drainage.

- Secure the dressing with adhesive tape or wrapping gauze, as appropriate.

Key Elements: Applying Wet-to-Damp Dressings

- Before applying the dressing, medicate the client as ordered.

- Maintain asepsis.

- Verify the ordered solution, and check agency policy about cleaning the wound.

- Remove the wet-to-damp dressing as quickly as possible, without moistening it.

- Assess the wound appearance and drainage accurately.

- Thoroughly saturate the mesh gauze with solution, and then wring out excess moisture.

- Make sure all depressions and grooves of the wound are packed with the gauze.

- Cover the wet dressings appropriately. Do not apply an airtight occlusive covering.

CLINICAL GUIDELINES

Postoperative Period
Assess to Determine

- *Vital signs: pulse, respirations, and blood pressure.* Compare results with data from the recovery room and preoperative baseline data. Many hospitals have postoperative routines for regular assessment of clients. In some agencies, assessments are made every 15 minutes until vital signs stabilize, every hour thereafter the same day, and every 4 hours for the next 2 days. Body temperature is usually assessed every 4 hours for the first few days. *It is very important that the assessments be made as frequently as the person's condition requires.* An elevated temperature, along with other signs, can indicate infection of the respiratory tract, urinary tract, or incision. A rapid, weak pulse and increased respiratory rate along with other signs can indicate infection, hemorrhage, or shock. A lowered blood pressure along with other signs can indicate hemorrhage, shock, or pulmonary embolism.

- *Skin color and temperature.* The color of the lips and nail beds are indicators of tissue perfusion (passage of blood through the capillaries). Pale, cyanotic, cool, and moist skin may be a sign of circulatory problems.

- *Level of consciousness.* During the early postoperative period, most clients are conscious but drowsy.

- *Bleeding.* Inspect the dressings for bleeding, and inspect the bedclothes underneath the client for pooled blood. When dressings are changed, inspect the wound for signs of localized infection.

- *Intravenous infusion.* Observe the type of solution, amount in the bottle, the drip rate, and the venipuncture site. Determine additional solutions ordered.

- *Patency of drainage tubes.* Note also the amount, color, consistency, and character of the drainage.

- *Fluid balance.* Measure the client's fluid intake and output for at least 2 days or until fluid balance is stable without an IV infusion.

- *Pain or discomfort and when the client last received an analgesic.* Note the location and type of pain, and determine the cause. Pain is usually greatest 12 to 36 hours after surgery, decreasing on the second or third day. Analgesics are usually administered every 3 or 4 hours the first day, and by the third day most clients require only oral analgesics. Signs of acute pain include pallor, perspiration, tension, and reluctance to perform deep-breathing and coughing exercises or to move or ambulate.

- *Any difficulties with voiding and/or bladder distention.*

- *Return of peristalsis.* Auscultate the client's abdomen to confirm the return of peristalsis. Note the passage of flatus and stool.

- *Tolerance of food and fluids ingested.*

Determine Clinical Signs
of Postoperative Complications

- *Pneumonia:* Elevated temperature, cough, expectoration of blood-tinged or purulent sputum, dyspnea, chest pain.

- *Atelectasis:* Marked dyspnea, cyanosis, pleural pain, tachycardia, increased respiratory rate, fever, productive cough, auscultatory crackling sounds.

- *Pulmonary embolism:* Sudden chest pain, shortness of breath, cyanosis, shock (tachycardia, low blood pressure).

- *Thrombophlebitis:* Aching, cramping pain; affected area is swollen, red, and hot to touch; vein feels hard; discomfort in calf when foot is dorsiflexed or when client walks (Homans' sign).

- *Thrombus or embolus:* Same as for pulmonary embolism; if lodged in heart or brain, assess cardiac or neurologic signs.

- *Urinary retention:* Fluid intake larger than output, inability to void or frequent voiding of small amounts, bladder distention, suprapubic discomfort, restlessness, bladder palpable above the pubic symphysis.

- *Urinary infection:* Burning sensation when voiding, urgency, cloudy urine, lower abdominal pain.

- *Constipation:* Absence of stool elimination, abdominal distention and discomfort.

- *Tympanites:* Obvious abdominal distention, abdominal discomfort (gas pains), absence of bowel sounds.

- *Wound infection:* Purulent exudate, redness, tenderness, elevated body temperature, wound odor.

- *Wound dehiscence:* Increased incision drainage; tissues underlying skin become visible along parts of the incision.

- *Wound evisceration:* Opening of incision and visible protrusion of organs.

Key Elements: Managing Gastrointestinal Suction

- Confirm the placement of the nasogastric tube before establishing suction.

- Place an air vent appropriately, and maintain its patency by injecting air.

- Test the functioning of the suction system before connecting it.

- Prevent kinks or blockages in the tubing.

- Keep all connections well sealed.

- Inspect the flow of gastric secretions into the drainage bottle.

- Clean the nares around the nasogastric tube at least every 3 hours.

- Provide mouth care.

Irrigations
- Obtain the physician's order if needed.

- Confirm the placement of the tube before irrigation.

- Reconnect the tube and attach it to suction following the procedure.

- Assess the amount and character of the drainage, client comfort, and abdominal distention.

Preventing Infections in the Home

- Wash your hands before handling foods, before eating, after toileting, before and after any required home care treatment, and after touching any body substances (eg, wound drainage).

- Keep your fingernails short, clean, and well-manicured to eliminate rough edges or hangnails, which can harbor microorganisms.

- Do not share personal care items: toothbrush, washcloths, and towels.

- Wash raw fruits and vegetables before eating them.

- Refrigerate all opened and nonpackaged foods.

- Clean used equipment (eg, emesis basin) with soap and water, and disinfect it with a chlorine bleach solution.

- Place contaminated dressings and other disposable items containing body fluids in moisture-proof plastic bags.

- Put used needles in a puncture-resistant container with a screw-top lid. Label so as not to discard in the garbage.

- Clean obviously soiled linen separately from other laundry. Rinse in cold water, wash in hot water if possible, and add a cup of bleach or Lysol to the wash.

- Avoid coughing, sneezing, or breathing directly on others. Cover the mouth and nose to prevent the transmission of airborne microorganisms.

- Be aware of any signs or symptoms of an infection, and report these immediately to your health care contact person.

- Maintain a sufficient fluid intake to promote urine production and output. This helps flush the bladder and urethra of microorganisms.

C. TEACHING AND LEARNING GUIDELINES

Teaching is a process designed to produce specific learning. The teaching/learning process involves dynamic interaction between the teacher and the learner. For teaching to be effective, trust must be established between the teacher and the learner, and communication must be open. Teaching is a five-step process analogous to the nursing process:

1. Collect data; analyze client's learning strengths and deficits.

2. Make educational diagnoses.

3. Prepare teaching plan.

4. Implement teaching plan.

5. Evaluate client learning (effectiveness of teaching process).

Nurses teach in a variety of ways and settings. Teaching may be planned, as in preoperative teaching. Teaching may also result during an interaction with a client. For example, when caring for a postoperative client, you find the client tense and in pain. Although the client has patient-controlled analgesia (PCA), you assess that the client doesn't understand how to use the pump. As part of your professional responsibilities, you must first make the client comfortable by administering the appropriate pain medicine and then teach the client how to utilize the PCA device.

Teaching can occur in many settings. In the hospital, teaching may be part of your daily client care. It may also be more formal, as in childbirth preparation classes or diabetes education classes. Teaching is a large part of home health and community health nursing. Teaching occurs in any location where nurses interact with clients.

When planning your client teaching, consider the following points:

- Learning requires energy and the ability to concentrate. Extreme anxiety or such physiologic factors as pain or sleep deprivation make it difficult for the client to learn. The nurse needs to consider the client's physical condition. The client, who has been medicated for pain, may or may not be ready for teaching. If the client is groggy from the medication, defer teaching; if, however, the pain medication has allowed the client to relax and become alert, this may be a good time to conduct a teaching session.

- Motivation is a powerful facilitator of learning. Clients who understand why they need to learn and who recognize the benefit of this knowledge are more likely to succeed. For example, the hazards of smoking are well known. Telling clients that quitting the habit will improve their health may not be sufficient; you must find out what is important to them so that the teaching is based on their learning needs, not yours.

- To maximize learning, create the best learning environment. It is often difficult to teach in a crowded hospital room. Roommates may have visitors or the television may be on, and privacy may not be possible. Attempt to modify the environment to promote learning. Plan to teach during quiet hours and when the client is comfortable and alert. Sometimes it is best to take the client to a quiet conference room.

- Establish rapport with the client before you begin instruction. Find out who the client is and what the client already knows. Build on the client's prior knowledge.

- Present your teaching in a form that the client can understand. Language and cultural differences may affect learning. For the client who speaks a different language, arrange translator services. Be careful when using family or support system members as translators. If it is important for the family to be part of the learning process, avoid asking them to act as translators; they may be so busy translating that they can't take in the information you present.

- Honor cultural differences. To establish rapport with the client and family, approach them with respect. Attempt to learn about the client's beliefs and values. Teaching that is in violation of cultural beliefs has little likelihood of succeeding. For more information on cultural issues, see Chapter 13 of *Fundamentals of Nursing*.

- Be certain to speak at the level the client can understand. Health care workers often speak in jargon. For example, a client may not understand what you mean when you say, "I'm going to straight cath you in order to get a sterile urine for C&S." You will need to explain this in terms that the client is familiar with and at the level that is appropriate for the client.

- Know your client. Choose your teaching strategy based on the client. Good teaching begins with client assessment. Determine what type of learner the client is, and orient your teaching according to this assessment. Is the client an auditory learner? If so, arrange a quiet time to talk. Is the client a visual learner? If so, discussion is not the best teaching strategy for this client. Instead, try drawings and pictures or video tapes. Is the client a hands-on learner, or is the material best presented in this fashion? Teaching a client how to self-administer an injection cannot be accomplished by merely talking about the technique. This type of teaching is best conducted by allowing the client to handle the syringe and medication.

- When teaching home care strategies, make sure you acquire adequate information about the home environment. Take the time to learn about the client so that the teaching is tailored to the client's situation. Suppose you are the hospital nurse caring for a client who has fallen and broken her hip. She has had surgery, and you are preparing her for discharge home. If the client is using a walker, can she get into a narrow bathroom with her walker? If she can't yet negotiate stairs, how will she manage at home if the bedroom and bath are upstairs and the kitchen downstairs? Interview the client so that your teaching can be geared to her situation. Maybe she needs a home health aide. You won't know if you don't ask, and if you don't ask the client may be back in the hospital with further problems.

- Make sure you are teaching the right person. Suppose, for example, that a beginning nursing student is caring for a newly diagnosed client with diabetes and gives him detailed instruction on modifying his diet. However, when making a home visit, the nurse finds that none of this information is being used. The teaching had been directed to the wrong person, because, as the client then informs the nurse, he does not do the shopping or the cooking. The nurse had failed to include the right person in her teaching. She should have asked the client's partner to participate in the diet instruction.

- Provide frequent feedback. Praise clients for what they have done well, and continue to work on areas that need improvement.

To summarize, effective teaching:

- holds the learner's interest.

- fosters a positive self-concept in the learner; learner believes learning is probable.

- supports the learner with positive reinforcement.

- makes partners of the learner and the teacher.

- is accurate and current.

- is appropriate for the learner's age, condition, and abilities.

- is optimistic, positive, and nonthreatening.

- is directed at helping the learner meet learning objectives.

- uses several methods of teaching to accommodate a variety of learning styles; provides learning opportunities through hearing, seeing, and doing.

- is cost-effective (the cost of the nurse's time spent teaching is less than the cost of treating health problems occurring when clients do not follow recommended treatments, fail to take medications correctly, or do not adapt lifestyle to changing health needs).

D. MEDICATIONS

Proper management of client medications is essential to safe patient care. A survey on use of drugs and medications, any allergies, or reports of problems with medications should be part of every nursing history. Safety consciousness should be uppermost in your mind when you administer medications. Always practice the "Five Rights":

- Right client
- Right medication
- Right dose
- Right time
- Right route

Check each medication thoroughly, and check the accuracy of the medication administration record (MAR) with the physician's order. A medication order must be complete. It must contain the client's name, the date, the medication, dose, route, method of administration, and signature of the prescriber. If any section of the order is unclear, difficult to read, or missing, contact the physician or advanced practice nurse. See Chapter 33 of *Fundamentals of Nursing* for a thorough discussion of medications, and remember, client safety must come first!

Check the medication against the order to be certain you are using the right medication. Many medications have similar names. Often a medication may be ordered in a trade name but be available in a generic form. Consult a drug guide to check for equivalency. With newer medications, you may need to consult a pharmacist for this type of information. After you have completed your preparation of the medication, check again for accuracy before you administer the medication to the client. Identify the client before administering any medication. Check the client's name band against the MAR. If the name band is missing, ask the client to identify himself or herself, or ask another nurse to verify the client's identity.

Your responsibility does not end once you administer the medication. A record must be kept of all medications administered. Promptly chart them after you administer them. When you get busy, it is tempting to postpone your charting. However, you run the risk that your preceptor will repeat the administration. Likewise, never chart a medication before giving it. When you chart, you are stating that you have prepared the medication and that the client has taken it. Too many things can go wrong if you prechart—the client may refuse, the client may be away from the unit at the prescribed time, or the client may even expire. Always chart that you have given the medication only after you have given it.

- Nurses who administer medications are responsible for their own actions. Question any order that you consider incorrect.

- Be knowledgeable about the medications you administer.

- Federal laws govern the uses of narcotics and barbiturates. Keep these medications in a locked place.

- Use only medications that are in a clearly labeled container.

- Return liquid medications that are cloudy or have changed color to the pharmacy.

- Do not leave medication at the bedside, with certain exceptions (eg, nitroglycerin, cough syrup). Determine agency policy.

- If a client vomits after taking an oral medication, report this to the nurse in charge.

- Take special precautions when administering certain medications; for example, have another nurse check the dosages of anticoagulants, insulin, and certain IV preparations.

- Most hospitals require new orders from the physician for the client's postsurgery care.

- When a medication is omitted for any reason, record the fact together with the reason.

- When a medication error is made, report it immediately to the nurse in charge.

The table on pages 212 and 213 includes common abbreviations used in medication orders.

Common Abbreviations Used in Medication Orders

Abbreviation	Explanation	Example of Administration Time
ac	before meals	0700, 1100, and 1700 hrs.
ad lib	freely, as desired	
agit	shake, stir	
aq	water	
aq dest	distilled water	
bid	twice a day	0900 and 2100 hrs.
c̄ (C)	with	
cap	capsule	
comp	compound	
dil	dilute	
elix	elixir	
g (G)	gram	
gr	grain	
gtt	drops	
h	an hour	
hs	at bedtime	
IM	intramuscular	
IV	intravenous	
m	minim	
mg	milligram	
mL (ml)	milliliter	
no. (#)	number	
OD	right eye	
OS (ol)	left eye	
OU	both eyes	
pc	after meals	0900, 1300, and 1900 hrs.
po	by mouth	
prn	when needed	

Abbreviation	Explanation	Example of Administration Time
q	every	
QAM (om)	every morning	1000 hrs.
qh (q1h)	every hour	
q2h	every 2 hrs.	0800, 1000, 1200 hrs., and so on
q3h	every 3 hrs.	0900, 1200, 1500 hrs., and so on
q4h	every 4 hrs.	1000, 1400, 1800 hrs., and so on
q6h	every 6 hrs.	0600, 1200, 1800, 2400 hrs.
qhs	every night at bedtime	
qid	four times a day	1000, 1400, 1800, 2200 hrs.
qod	every other day	0900 hrs. on odd dates
qs	sufficient quantity	
Rx	take, prescription	
s̄ (S)	without	
sc	subcutaneous	
sig (s)	label	
sos	if necessary	
ss (s̄s̄)	one half	
sup (supp)	suppository	
susp	suspension	
tid	three times a day	1000, 1400, and 1800 hrs
Tr (tinct)	tincture	

Converting Weights and Measures Among Systems

When preparing client medications, a nurse may need to convert weights or volumes from one system to another. As an example, the pharmacy may dispense milligrams or grams of chloral hydrate, yet the nurse must administer an order that reads chloral hydrate grains viiss. To prepare the correct dose, the nurse must convert from the apothecaries' to the metric system. To give clients a useful, realistic measure for home use, the nurse may have to convert from the apothecaries' or metric system to the household system. All conversions are approximate, that is, not totally precise.

For example, a physician orders morphine gr ¼. The medication is available only in milligrams. The nurse knows that 1 mg = ¹⁄₆₀ gr or 60 mg = 1 grain. To convert the ordered dose to milligrams, the nurse calculates as follows:

$$\text{If } 60 \text{ mg} = 1 \text{ gr}$$

$$\text{Then } x \text{ mg} = \tfrac{1}{4} \text{ gr } (0.25 \text{ gr})$$

$$x = \frac{60 \times 0.25}{1}$$

$$x = 15 \text{ mg}$$

Calculating Dosages

There are several formulas that can be used to calculate drug dosages. One formula uses ratios:

$$\frac{\text{dose on hand}}{\text{quantity on hand}} = \frac{\text{desired dose}}{\text{quantity desired } (x)}$$

For example, erythromycin 500 mg is ordered. It is supplied in a liquid form containing 250 mg in 5 mL. To calculate the dosage, use the formula:

$$\frac{\text{dose on hand (250)}}{\text{quantity on hand (5 mL)}} = \frac{\text{desired dose (500 mg)}}{\text{quantity desired } (x)}$$

Then, cross-multiply:

$$250\,x = 5\text{ mL} \times 500\text{ mg}$$
$$x = \frac{5\text{ mL} \times 500\text{ mg}}{250\text{ mg}}$$
$$x = 10\text{ mg}$$

Therefore, the dose ordered is 10 mL.

Another method for dosage calculation is:

$$\text{amount to administer } (x) =$$
$$\frac{\text{desired dose}}{\text{dose on hand} \times \text{quantity on hand}}$$

For example, heparin is often distributed in large vials and prepared dilutions of 10,000 units per mL. If the order calls for 5000 units, the nurse can calculate using the formula above:

$$x = \frac{5000}{10{,}000} \times 1$$

$$x = \frac{1}{2} \times \text{mL}$$

Therefore, the nurse injects 0.5 mL for a 5000 unit dose.

Injection Techniques

Review the illustrations on pages 216–222 for injection sites, types of injections, and injection techniques.

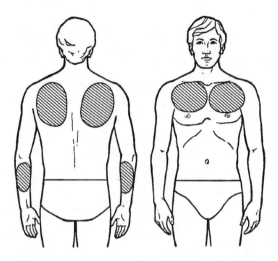

Body sites commonly used for intradermal injections.

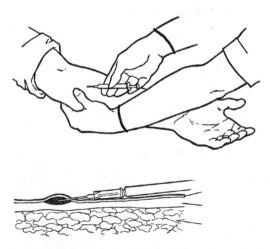

For an intradermal injection: **A,** the needle enters the skin at a 15 degree angle; and **B,** the medication forms a bleb under the epidermis.

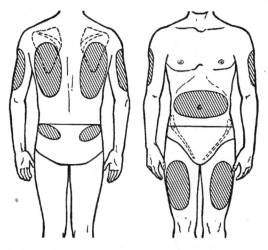

Body sites commonly used for subcutaneous injections.

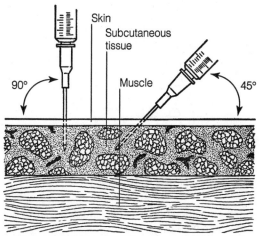

Inserting a needle into the subcutaneous tissue using 90 degree and 45 degree angles.

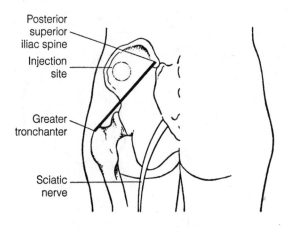

One method of establishing the dorsogluteal site for an intramuscular injection.

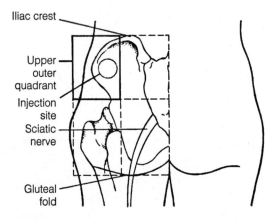

Another method of establishing the dorsogluteal site for an intramuscular injection.

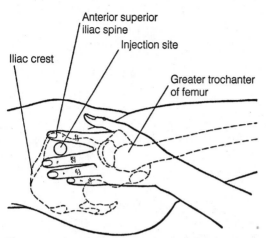

The ventrogluteal site for an intramuscular injection.

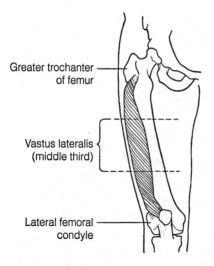

The vastus lateralis site for an intramuscular injection.

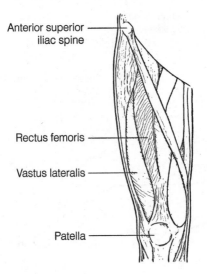

The rectus femoris muscle of the upper right thigh, used for intramuscular injections.

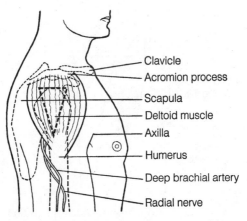

The deltoid muscle of the upper arm, used for intramuscular injections.

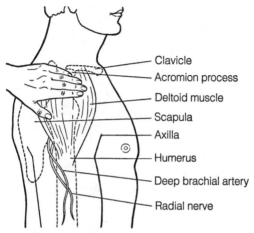

- Clavicle
- Acromion process
- Deltoid muscle
- Scapula
- Axilla
- Humerus
- Deep brachial artery
- Radial nerve

A method of establishing the deltoid muscle for an intramuscular injection.

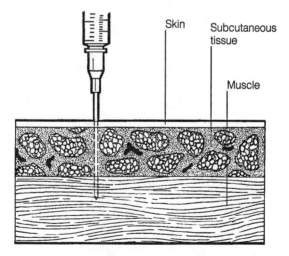

Skin Subcutaneous tissue

Muscle

An intramuscular needle inserted into the muscle layer.

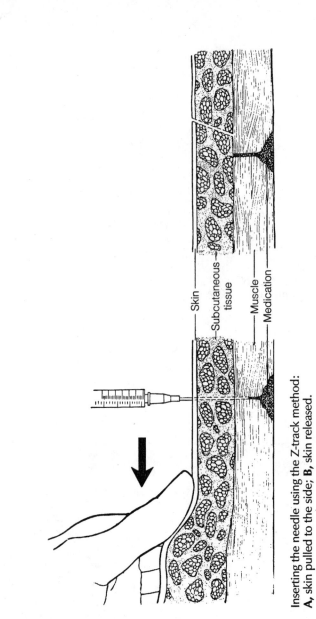

Inserting the needle using the Z-track method:
A, skin pulled to the side; **B,** skin released.

Skin

Subcutaneous tissue

Muscle

Medication

UNIT 4

Documentation and Evaluation

A. Charting Guidelines
B. SOAP Format
C. Evaluation

A. CHARTING GUIDELINES

Charting is a written method of conveying client information, nursing assessments and interventions, and client response to care. For a thorough discussion of documentation and reporting, review Chapter 21 of *Fundamentals of Nursing*. The following list of guidelines can help you chart accurately.

- Make sure the nursing record is stamped with client's name before you begin writing.

- Write legibly; print if necessary. Always write in permanent ink.

- Begin each entry with the time and date of the recording. End each entry with a signature that consists of your first initial, last name, and abbreviated title.

- Never erase or use white-out. Cross through a mistake with a single line, write the word "mistaken entry" above it, and initial the change.

- If a blank space appears in a notation, draw a line through the blank space so that no additional information can be recorded at any other time or by any other person.

- Write your notes as soon as possible after giving nursing care.

- Be precise. State your assessments objectively. Report the client's subjective opinions by quoting directly. Avoid using words that convey judgment or inference—just state the facts.

- Use only commonly accepted abbreviations, symbols, and terms specified by the agency.

- Record your teaching.

- Remember that from a legal perspective, if you didn't chart it, you didn't do it!

Essential Client Information

The following may assist you in selecting essential client information to record. Note that you should emphasize data that denote a change in the client's health status or behavior and data that indicate a deviation from what is usually expected.

1. Any behavior changes, for example,

   - indications of strong emotions, such as anxiety or fear.

   - marked changes in mood.

   - a change in level of consciousness, such as stupor.

   - regression in relationships with family or friends.

2. Any changes in physical function, such as

   - loss of balance.

   - loss of strength.

   - difficulty hearing or seeing.

3. Any physical sign or symptom that

- is severe, such as severe pain.

- tends to recur or persist.

- deviates from normal, such as elevated body temperature.

- gets worse, such as gradual weight loss.

- indicates faulty health habits, such as lice on the scalp.

- is a known danger signal, such as a lump in the breast.

4. Any nursing interventions provided, such as

- medications administered.

- therapies.

- activities of daily living, if agency policy dictates.

- teaching clients self-care.

5. Select data gathered from visits by a physician or other members of the health team.

B. SOAP FORMAT

SOAP is an acronym for subjective data, objective data, assessment, and planning. The SOAP format originated with the problem-oriented medical record (POMR) but is used increasingly in many different types of records. The acronyms SOAPIE and SOAPIER refer to formats that also include implementation, evaluation, and revision. Many agencies use only the SOAP format. A more recent format is the APIE (assessment, plan, implementation, and evaluation), which condenses the client data into fewer statements. In APIE, the assessment combines the nursing diagnosis; the plan combines the nursing actions with the expected outcomes; and the implementation and evaluation are the same. The following are examples of a nurse's progress notes using the SOAP, SOAPIER, and APIE formats.

Nursing Progress Notes

SOAP Format

2/13/04 #5 Generalized pruritus
1400
S— "My skin is itchy on my back and arms, and it's been like this for a week."
O— Skin appears clear; no rash or irritations noted. Marks where client has scratched noted on left and right forearms. Allergic to elastoplast but has not been in contact.
No previous history of pruritus.
A— High risk for infection related to scratching secondary to pruritus.
P— Instructed to not scratch skin.
— Applied calamine lotion to back and arms at 1430 h.
— Cut fingernails.

SOAPIER Format

2/13/04 #5 Generalized pruritus
1400
S— "My skin is itchy on back and arms and it's been like this for a week."
O— Skin appears clear; no rash or irritation noted. Marks where client has scratched noted on left and right forearms. Allergic to elastoplast but has not been in contact.
No previous history of pruritus.
A— High risk for infection.
P— Instruct not to scratch skin.
— Apply calamine lotion as necessary.
— Cut nails to avoid scratches.

APIE Format

2/13/04 #5 Generalized pruritus
1400
A— High risk for infection (scratching). States, "My skin is itchy on my back and arms, and it's been like this for a week."
Skin appears clear.
— No rash or irritations noted. Marks where client has scratched noted on left and right forearms. Allergic to elastoplast but has not been in contact.
No previous history of pruritus.
P— Instruct not to scratch skin.
— Apply calamine lotion as necessary.
— Cut nails to avoid scratches.

SOAP Format

— Assess further to determine if recurrence associated with specific drugs or foods.
— Refer to physician and pharmacist for assessment.

Tom Ritchie, RN

SOAPIER Format

— Assess further to determine if recurrence associated with specific drugs or foods.
— Refer to physician and pharmacist for assessment.
I— Instructed not to scratch skin. Applied calamine lotion to back and arms at 1430 h. Assisted to cut fingernails. Notified physician and pharmacist of problem.

1600
E— States, "I'm still itchy. That lotion didn't help."
R— Remove calamine lotion and apply hydrocortisone ungt. as ordered.

Tom Ritchie, RN

APIE Format

— Assess further to determine if recurrence associated with specific drugs or foods.
— Refer to doctor and pharmacist for assessment.
I— Instructed not to scratch skin. Applied calamine lotion to back and arms at 1430 h. Assisted to cut fingernails. Notified physician and pharmacist of problem.
E— States, "I'm still itchy. That lotion didn't help."

Tom Ritchie, RN

C. EVALUATION

Evaluation is the final phase of the nursing process, in which the nurse determines the client's progress toward goal/outcome achievement and the effectiveness of the nursing care plan. Evaluating

- is determining whether or to what degree client goals have been met.

- may be ongoing, intermittent, or terminal.

- is purposeful and organized.

- uses desired outcomes formulated in the planning phase as criteria for evaluating client progress.

Glossary

abdominal paracentesis removal of fluid from the peritoneal cavity

abduction movement of a body part away from the midline of the body

abrasion scraping away of a structure, such as the skin or teeth

abscess a localized collection of pus and disintegrating body cells

absorption (of drug) the process by which a drug passes into the blood stream

acapnia a decreased level of carbon dioxide in the blood

acidosis (acidemia) a condition that occurs with increases in blood carbonic acid or with decreases in blood bicarbonate; arterial blood pH below 7.35

acromion (acromial process) the lateral projection of the scapula extending over the shoulder joint

active exercise exercise carried out by the client, who supplies the energy to move the body parts

activities of daily living (ADLs) the tasks of daily life, such as eating, bathing, and dressing

acute sharp or severe; describing a severe condition with a sudden onset and short course (as opposed to chronic)

adduction movement of a body part toward the midline of the body

adipose fat; of a fatty nature

adventitious breath sounds abnormal breath sounds

albuminuria the presence of albumin in the urine

aldosterone a hormone produced by the adrenal cortex that regulates the level of sodium in the body

alkalosis (alkalemia) a condition that occurs with increases in blood bicarbonate or decreases in blood carbonic acid; arterial blood pH above 7.45

alopecia abnormal loss of hair

alveolus a small saclike dilation or cavity in the body

ampule a small, sealed glass flask, usually designed to hold a single dose of medication

analgesic a medication used to decrease pain

anaphylaxis (anaphylactic shock, anaphylactic reaction) a severe allergic reaction

anasarca generalized edema throughout the body

anemia a condition in which the blood is deficient in red blood cells or hemoglobin

anesthesia loss of sensation or feeling; induced loss of the sense of pain

aneurysm dilation of the wall of an artery or vein

angiography a diagnostic procedure allowing x-ray visualization of the vascular system after injection of a radiopaque dye

anorexia lack of appetite

anoxemia a condition in which the level of oxygen in the blood is below normal

anoxia systemic absence or reduction of oxygen in the body tissues below physiologic levels

anterior toward or at the front of

antibiotic a substance that has the capacity to inhibit the growth of or kill microorganisms

antibody (immunoglobulin) a protective substance produced in the body to counteract antigens

antidiuretic hormone (ADH) a hormone that is stored and released by the posterior pituitary gland and that controls water reabsorption from the kidney tubules; also referred to as vasopressin

antigen a substance capable of inducing the formation of antibodies

antipyretic a substance that is effective in reducing fever

antiseptic an agent that inhibits the growth of some microorganisms

anuria the failure of the kidneys to produce urine, resulting in total lack of urination or output of less than 100 mL per day in an adult

apathy lack of interest or feeling

aphasia the inability to communicate by speech, signs, or writing, resulting from an injury or disease

apical pulse the central pulse, located at the apex of the heart

apical-radial pulse measurement of the apical beat and the radial pulse

apnea cessation of breathing

apneustic breathing prolonged, gasping inspiration followed by a very short, usually inefficient expiration

approximate to bring close together (referring to wound or incision edges)

areflexia absence of reflexes

arrhythmia an irregular cardiac rhythm

arteriosclerosis a condition in which the walls of the arteries become hardened, thickened, and less compliant

ascites the accumulation of fluid in the abdominal cavity

asepsis freedom from infection or infectious material

asphyxia a condition resulting from a lack of oxygen

aspirate to remove gases or fluids from a cavity by using suction

astringent an agent that causes contraction or shrinkage of tissue; usually applied topically

ataxia failure of muscle coordination

atelectasis collapse of lung tissue

atony lack of normal muscle tone

atrophy a wasting away or decrease in size of a cell, tissue, body organ, or muscle

auscultation the practice of examining the body by listening to body sounds

axilla the armpit (plural: axillae)

axillary line an imaginary line extending vertically from the anterior fold of the axilla

bacteriuria bacteria in the urine

barium a metallic element commonly used in solution as a contrast medium for x-ray filming of the gastrointestinal tract

barium enema x-ray filming of the large intestine using a contrast medium; also called a lower gastrointestinal series

barium swallow x-ray filming of the esophagus, stomach, and duodenum; also referred to as an upper gastrointestinal series

barrel chest a chest shape in which the ratio of the anteroposterior diameter to the lateral diameter is 1 to 1

basal metabolic rate (BMR) the rate of energy utilization in the body required to maintain body functions at rest

Beau's line a deep line visible across a nail after its growth has been halted and then renewed

bilateral affecting two sides

bilirubin orange or yellow pigment in the bile

binder a type of bandage applied to large body areas, such as the abdomen or chest

biopsy the removal and examination of tissue from the living body

bleb (wheal) a small, smooth, slightly raised area on the skin, usually filled with fluid

borborygmi abnormally intense and frequent bowel sounds

brachial pulse a pulse located on the inner side of the biceps muscle just below the axilla; usually palpated medially in the antecubital space

bradycardia an abnormally slow heart rate, below 60 beats per minute in an adult

bradypnea abnormally slow respiration, usually fewer than 10 respirations per minute

bromhidrosis foul-smelling perspiration

bronchial sounds normal loud, harsh, hollow blowing sounds heard by auscultation over the trachea and major bronchi

bronchodilator an agent that dilates the bronchi of the lungs

bronchophony an increase in vocal resonance; an abnormal voice sound heard on auscultation of the chest wall

bronchopneumonia an infection that originates in the bronchi and involves patches of lung tissue

bronchoscope a lighted instrument used to visualize the bronchi of the lungs

bronchoscopy visual examination of the bronchi using a bronchoscope

bronchovesicular sounds combination of bronchial and vesicular sounds heard by auscultation over parts of the chest where a bronchus is near lung tissue

bruit abnormal blowing, swishing, or rippling sounds heard during auscultation

bruxism grinding of the teeth during sleep

bubbling gurgling sounds produced as air passes through moist secretions in the respiratory tract

buccal pertaining to the cheek

buffer an agent or system that tends to maintain constancy of or that prevents changes in the chemical concentration of a substance

bulimia an uncontrollable compulsion to consume enormous amounts of food and then expel the food by self-induced vomiting or by taking laxatives

calculus a stone composed of minerals that is formed in the body, for example, a renal calculus formed in the kidney

cannula a tube with a lumen (channel), which is inserted into a cavity or duct and is often fitted with a trocar during insertion

canthus the angle formed by the upper and lower eyelids; each eye has an inner and an outer canthus

cardiac arrest the cessation of heart function

cardiac output the amount of blood ejected from the heart per minute by ventricular contraction; it is the stroke volume times the heart rate per minute

cardiopulmonary resuscitation (CPR) artificial stimulation of the heart and lungs; also referred to as basic life support (BLS)

caries decay of a tooth or bone

carina the ridge or junction where the main bronchi meet the trachea

carminative an agent that prevents the formation of gas in the colon

carotid arteries major arteries lying on either side of the trachea and larynx

cataract opacity of the lens of the eye or its capsule

cathartic (laxative) a drug that induces evacuation of feces from the large intestine

catheter a tube of plastic, rubber, metal, or other material used to remove or inject fluids into a cavity, such as the bladder

caudal anesthetic an anesthetic injected into the caudal canal, below the spinal cord

cellulitis inflammation of cellular tissue

centigrade (Celsius) a thermometer scale used to measure heat; the freezing point of water is 0C, and the boiling point is 100C

central venous pressure (CVP) a measurement of the pressure of the blood, in millimeters of water, within the vena cava or the right atrium of the heart

cephalocaudal proceeding in the direction from head to toe

cerebral death death that occurs when the cerebral cortex is irreversibly destroyed

cerebrospinal fluid fluid contained within the four ventricles of the brain, the subarachnoid space, and the central canal of the spinal cord

cerumen waxlike material found in the external auditory canal

chancre a papular lesion (sore) occurring at the primary site of infection in some diseases; the primary sore of syphilis

cheilosis cracks or scaling at the corners of the lips

Cheyne-Stokes respirations rhythmic waxing and waning of respirations from very deep breathing to very shallow breathing with periods of temporary apnea; often associated with cardiac failure, increased intracranial pressure, or brain damage

chill shivering and shaking of the body with involuntary contractions of the voluntary muscles

cholangiogram an x-ray film of the biliary tract taken after the injection of a dye

cholecystogram an x-ray film of the gallbladder after the ingestion of a contrast dye; also called *oral cholecystography*

cholesterol a lipid that does not contain fatty acid but possesses many of the chemical and physical properties of other lipids

chronic persisting over a long time

chyme semifluid material produced by gastric digestion of food in the stomach; it is found in the small and large intestines

cicatrix scar

cilia hairlike projections from cells, for example, cells of the mucous membrane of the respiratory tract

circulatory overload a state of increased blood volume

circumduction movement of the distal part of a bone in a circle, with the proximal end remaining fixed

clean technique a technique that maintains an area or articles free from infectious agents

closed wound a wound in which there is no break in the skin

clubbing (of nails) an elevation of the proximal aspect of the nail and softening of the nail bed

coagulate to clot

cochlea a tubular structure in the inner ear that contains the organ for hearing

cognitive referring to intellectual processes such as remembering, thinking, perceiving, abstracting, and generalizing

colic paroxysmal intestinal cramplike pain

collagen a protein found in connective tissue; a whitish protein substance that adds tensile strength to a wound

colonoscope a lighted instrument used to visualize the interior of the colon

colonoscopy visual examination of the interior of the colon with a colonoscope

colostomy an artificial abdominal opening into the colon (large bowel)

comatose a state of unconsciousness in which the person shows no response to maximum painful stimuli, absence of reflexes, and absence of muscle tone in the extremities

commode a portable chairlike structure used as a toilet

communicable disease (infectious disease) a disease that can spread from one person to another

compliance in learning, an individual's desire to learn and act on the learning; in drug therapy, the act of carefully following the prescription; of the arteries, distensibility or the ability to contract and expand

congenital existing at, and often before, birth

conjunctiva the delicate membrane that covers the eyeball and lines the eyelids

conjunctivitis inflammation of the conjunctiva

consciousness a person's normal state of awareness of the environment, self, and others

consensual reaction (of the eyes) a reaction in which one pupil constricts quickly in response to a bright light and the other pupil constricts also, but more slowly

constipation passage of small, dry, hard stool or passage of no stool for an abnormally long time

contaminated possessing disease-producing microorganisms

contracture permanent shortening of a muscle and subsequent shortening of tendons and ligaments

contusion a closed wound that occurs as a result of a blow from a blunt instrument; a bruise

cordotomy (chordotomy) surgical severing of the spinothalamic portion of the anterolateral tract of the spinal cord, usually for the purpose of relieving pain

core temperature temperature of the deep structures of the body

cornea the transparent covering of the anterior eye that connects with the sclera

costal angle the angle formed between the ribs and the sternum

costal (thoracic) breathing breathing using chiefly the intercostal muscles

costovertebral angle the angle formed by a rib and the spine

counterirritant an agent that produces an irritation with the intent of relieving some other problem

crackles (rales) rattling or bubbling breath sounds generally heard on inspiration

creatinine a nitrogenous waste that is excreted in the urine

Credé's maneuver manual exertion of pressure on the bladder to force urine out

crepitus (crepitation) skeletal: a grating sound caused by bone fragments rubbing together; respiratory: a dry, crackling sound like that of crumpled cellophane, produced by air in the subcutaneous tissue or by air moving through fluid in the alveoli of the lungs

culture in microbiology, the cultivation of microorganisms or cells in a special growth medium

curet a spoon-shaped instrument used for removing material from a body cavity

cyanosis bluish discoloration of the skin, nail beds, and mucous membranes, due to reduced oxygen in the blood

cyst an enclosed cavity or sac lined by epithelium and containing liquid or semisolid material

cystitis inflammation of the urinary bladder

cystoscope a lighted instrument used to visualize the interior of the urinary bladder

cystoscopy visual examination of the urinary bladder with a cystoscope

cytology the study of the origin, structure, function, and pathology of cells

dacryocystitis inflammation of the lacrimal sac

debride to remove foreign and dying tissue from a wound so that healthy tissue is exposed

decubitus ulcer an ulcer of the skin and underlying tissues produced by prolonged pressure; also known as *pressure sore*

defecation expulsion of feces from the rectum and anus

dehiscence a splitting open or rupture

dehydration insufficient fluid in the body

dementia decline in memory and other cognitive abilities

demineralization excessive loss of minerals or inorganic salts

dependent edema edema that collects in the lower parts of the body, where hydrostatic pressure is greatest

dermatitis inflammation of the skin

dermatologic preparation a medication applied to the skin

dermis (corium) true skin, containing blood vessels, nerves, hair follicles, and glands

detrusor muscle the three layers of smooth muscle that make up the urinary bladder

dextrose a sugar; also called *glucose*

diagnosis a statement or conclusion concerning the nature of some phenomenon

diaphoresis profuse sweating

diaphragmatic (abdominal) breathing breathing that chiefly involves movement of the diaphragm and the abdomen

diarrhea defecation of liquid feces and increased frequency of defecation

diastole the period when the ventricles of the heart are relaxed

diastolic pressure the pressure of the blood against the arterial walls when the ventricles of the heart are at rest

digital performed with the finger

disorientation a state of mental confusion; loss of bearings, time, and place

distal farthest from the point of reference

distention (abdominal) *see* **tympanites**

diuresis *see* **polyuria**

diuretic an agent that increases the production of urine

dorsal of, toward, or at the back

dorsal flexion movement of the ankle so that the toes point up

dorsalis pedis pulse a pulse located on the instep of the foot

dorsal recumbent position a back-lying position with the head and shoulders slightly elevated

drainage a discharge from a wound or cavity

drug interaction the beneficial or harmful interaction of one drug with another drug

drug tolerance a condition in which successive increases in the dosage of a drug are required to maintain a given therapeutic effect

drug toxicity the quality of a drug that exerts a deleterious effect on an organism or tissue

dullness (in percussion) decreased resonance or percussion sound that occurs over dense tissue or large amounts of fluid

dysmenorrhea painful menstruation

dyspepsia indigestion

dysphagia difficulty or inability to swallow

dysphasia difficulty speaking

dysphoria a feeling of disquiet, restlessness, anxiety, depression

dyspnea difficult and labored breathing in which the client has a persistent unsatisfied need for air

dysrhythmia an irregular cardiac rhythm

dysuria painful or difficult urination

ecchymosis a blotchy area of discoloration of the skin; a bruise

edema excess interstitial fluid

effluent urine or feces discharged through a stoma

egophony a type of bronchophony in which the voice has a nasal, bleating quality

electrocardiogram (ECG, EKG) a graph of the electric activity of the heart

electroencephalogram (EEG) a graph of the electric activity of the brain

electrolyte ionized salts found in cells, tissue fluids, and blood

embolus a blood clot (or a substance, such as air) that has moved from its place of origin and is obstructing the circulation in a blood vessel (plural: *emboli*)

emollient an agent that soothes and softens skin or mucous membrane; often an oily substance

emphysema a chronic obstructive lung disorder in which the terminal bronchioles become distended and plugged with mucus

emulsion a preparation in which one liquid is distributed throughout another

endemic present in a particular population or community all the time

endogenous developing from within

endoscope a lighted instrument used to visualize the interior of a hollow organ

endothelium the layer of endothelial cells lining the blood vessels, cavities of the heart, and serous cavities

endotracheal tube a tube inserted into the trachea

enema a solution injected into the rectum and the sigmoid colon

enteric referring to the small intestines

enteric-coated surrounded with a special coating used for tablets and capsules that prevents release of the drug until it is in the intestines

enteric feeding a feeding administered directly into the small intestine through a tube

enteritis inflammation of the small intestine

enterostomal therapist a person who specializes in ostomy care

enterostomy an opening through the abdominal wall into the intestines

enzyme a biologic catalyst that induces chemical reactions

epidemic the occurrence of a disease in many people at the same time or in rapid succession in an area

epidermis the outermost, nonvascular layer of skin

epistaxis nosebleed

eructation ejection of gas from the stomach (belching)

erythema redness that is associated with a variety of rashes

erythrocyte red blood cell

erythropoiesis the formation of red blood cells

eschar a slough of dried plasma proteins and dead cells; often produced by a burn, corrosive application, or gangrene

esophagoscopy visual examination of the interior of the esophagus with a lighted instrument

etiology cause

eupnea normal respiration that is quiet, rhythmic, and effortless

evisceration removal of or spilling out of the internal organs

exanthema skin rash

excise to cut off or out

excoriation abrasion of the superficial layers of the skin

excretion elimination of waste products from the body

exogenous developing from without

expectorate to cough and spit up mucus or other materials

expiratory reserve volume the maximum amount of air exhaled after a normal exhalation

extension increasing the angle of a joint (between two bones); the act of straightening

external cardiac massage rhythmic massage of the heart muscle over the sternum

extracellular outside the cells

extracellular fluid (ECF) fluid found outside the body cells

extravasation the escape of blood from a vessel into body tissues

exudate material, such as fluid and cells, that has escaped from blood vessels and is deposited in tissues or on tissue surfaces during the inflammatory process

febrile pertaining to a fever; feverish

fecal impaction a mass of hardened feces in the rectum

fecal incontinence inability to control the passage of feces through the anus

feces (stool) body wastes and undigested food eliminated from the rectum

femoral pulse the pulse found in the groin at the midpoint of the inguinal ligament

fenestrated perforated to provide a window or opening

fever elevated body temperature

fibrillation involuntary contractions of a muscle; cardiac arrhythmia characterized by extremely rapid, irregular, and ineffective contractions of the atria or ventricles

fibrinous exudate exudate containing large amounts of fibrin

first intention healing primary healing of a wound, which occurs when the tissue surfaces have been approximated

fistula an abnormal communication or passage, usually between two organs or between an organ and the body surface

flaccid weak or lax

flaccid paralysis impaired muscle function with loss of muscle tone

flail chest a condition of the chest wall caused by two or more rib fractures resulting in paradoxical breathing

flatness (in percussion) absence of resonance; extreme dullness

flatulence the presence of excessive amounts of gas in the stomach or intestines

flatus gas or air normally present in the stomach or intestines

flexion decreasing the angle of a joint (between two bones); the act of bending

flowsheet a record used to chart the progress of specific or specialized data, such as vital signs, fluid balance, or routine medications

fluoroscope a device for examining internal structures using roentgen rays

fluoroscopy an examination using a fluoroscope

flushing (of the skin) transient redness of the skin, often of the face and neck; it may be generalized or restricted to a particular area

footdrop plantar flexion of the foot with permanent contracture of the gastrocnemius (calf) muscle and tendon

forceps an instrument with two blades and a handle used to grasp sterile supplies and to compress or grasp tissues

foreskin a covering fold of skin over the glans of the penis; also called the *prepuce*

formulary a collection or list of prescriptions and formulas

Fowler's position a bed-sitting position with the head of the bed raised to 45 degrees

fracture a break in the continuity of bone

fremitus vibration perceptible on palpation

frenulum a fold of mucous membrane that attaches the tongue to the floor of the mouth; a fold on the lower surface of the glans penis that connects it with the prepuce

friction rub *see* **pleural rub**

funnel chest a congenital defect in which the sternum is depressed and the anteroposterior diameter of the chest is narrowed

gait the way a person walks

gastric pertaining to the stomach

gastrocolic reflex increased peristalsis of the colon after food has entered the stomach

gastroenteritis inflammation of the stomach and the intestines

gastroscope a lighted instrument used to visualize the interior of the stomach

gastroscopy visual examination of the stomach with a gastroscope

gastrostomy a surgical opening that leads through the abdomen directly into the stomach

gauge (of a needle) the diameter of the shaft of a needle

gavage administration of nourishment to the stomach through a nasogastric or orogastric tube; tube feeding

generic name a drug name not protected by trademark and usually describing the chemical structure of the drug

genupectoral position a position in which the weight is borne by the knees and chest and the body is at a 90-degree angle to the hips; also called *knee-chest position*

gingiva the gum tissue

gingivitis inflammation of the gums

glans penis the cap-shaped, expansive structure at the end of the penis

glaucoma an eye disease characterized by an increase in intraocular pressure that produces changes in the optic disc and the field of vision

glomerular filtrate fluid formed in the nephron of the kidney that is similar to plasma in composition; the precursor of urine

glossitis inflammation of the tongue

glottis the vocal apparatus of the larynx

glucose a monosaccharide occurring in food

glycogen the chief carbohydrate stored in the body, particularly in the liver and muscles

glycosuria the presence of glucose in the urine; glucosuria

gonorrhea a sexually transmitted disease due to *Neisseria gonorrhoeae* infection

gout a condition characterized by excessive uric acid in the blood

granulation tissue young connective tissue with new capillaries formed in the wound-healing process

gustatory referring to the sense of taste

half-life (of drug) the time interval required for the body's elimination processes to reduce the concentration of the drug in the body by one half

halitosis bad breath

hallux valgus bunion or lateral deviation of the big toe

haustrum a saclike formation of a part of the colon, produced by contraction of both the longitudinal and the circular muscles (plural: *haustra*)

Heimlich maneuver subdiaphragmatic abdominal thrusts used to clear an obstructed airway

hemangioma a large, persistent, bright red or dark purple vascular area of the skin

hematemesis the vomiting of blood

hematocrit the percentage of red blood cell mass in proportion to whole blood

hematoma a collection of blood in a tissue, organ, or body space due to a break in the wall of a blood vessel

hematuria the presence of blood in the urine

hemiplegia the loss of movement on one side of the body

hemoglobin the red pigment in red blood cells that carries oxygen

hemoglobinuria the presence of hemoglobin in the urine

hemolysis rupture of red blood cells

hemopneumothorax a collection of blood and air or gas in the pleural cavity

hemoptysis the presence of blood in the sputum

hemorrhage bleeding; the escape of blood from the blood vessels

hemorrhoids distended veins in the anus and rectum

hemosiderosis deposition of iron in the skin, liver, spleen, and other organs

hemothorax a collection of blood in the pleural cavity

heparin a substance that prevents coagulation of blood

heparin lock an indwelling intravenous catheter attached to a plastic tube with a sealed injection tip

hernia protrusion of an organ or tissue through an opening in the wall of the cavity that usually contains it

hesitancy (of urination) delay and difficulty initiating voiding

high-Fowler's position a bed-sitting position in which the head of the bed is elevated 90 degrees

hirsutism abnormal hairiness, particularly in women

Homans' sign calf pain produced by dorsiflexion of the foot, an early sign of venous thrombosis

homeostasis tendency of the body to maintain a state of balance or equilibrium while continually changing

humidifier a device that adds water vapor to inspired air

hydration the addition of water to a substance or tissue

hydrocephalus a disease process resulting in excessive cerebrospinal fluid within the ventricles of the brain

hydrocortisone an adrenocorticosteroid produced by the adrenal glands or produced synthetically; also called *cortisol*

hyperalgesia extreme sensitivity to pain

hyperalimentation *see* **total parenteral nutrition**

hypercalcemia excessive calcium in the blood plasma

hypercalciuria excessive calcium in the urine

hypercarbia (hypercapnia) accumulation of carbon dioxide in the blood

hyperchloremia an excess of serum chloride

hyperemia increased blood flow to an area

hyperextension further extension between two bones or stretching out of a joint

hyperglycemia an increased concentration of glucose in the blood

hyperhidrosis excessive perspiration

hyperkalemia excessive potassium in the blood

hyperlipidemia elevated concentration of lipids in the plasma

hypermagnesemia excessive magnesium in the blood plasma

hypernatremia an elevated level of sodium in the blood plasma

hyperphosphatemia increased phosphorus levels in the blood plasma

hyperplasia an abnormal increase in the number of normal cells in a tissue or an organ

hyperpnea an increase in the rate of breathing or an increase in depth of respirations

hyperpyrexia an extremely elevated body temperature

hyperreflexia an exaggeration of the reflexes

hyperresonance a sound that is lower-pitched than resonance; booming sound

hypersensitivity an exaggerated response of the body to a foreign substance

hypersomnia excessive sleep

hypertension an abnormally high blood pressure

hyperthermia an abnormally high body temperature, sometimes induced as a therapeutic measure

hypertonicity excessive muscle tone or activity

hypertonic solution a fluid possessing a greater concentration of solutes than plasma

hypertrophy an increase in size of a cell, tissue, or body organ, such as a muscle

hyperventilation an increase in the amount of air entering the lungs, characterized by deep, rapid breaths

hypervolemia an abnormal increase in the body's blood volume; circulatory overload

hypnotic (drug) a drug that induces sleep

hypoalbuminemia reduction in the level of albumin in the blood

hypocalcemia decreased calcium in the blood plasma

hypocarbia (hypocapnia) depressed level of carbon dioxide in the blood

hypochloremia a reduced concentration of chlorides in the blood plasma

hypoglycemia a reduced amount of glucose in the blood

hypokalemia potassium deficit in the blood plasma

hypomagnesemia low magnesium in the blood plasma

hyponatremia an abnormally low amount of sodium in the blood plasma

hypophosphatemia phosphorus deficiency in the blood

hypopnea decreased rate and depth of respiration

hypoproteinemia decreased amount of protein in the blood plasma

hypostatic pneumonia an infection of lung tissue resulting from poor circulation or stagnation of secretions

hypotension an abnormally low blood pressure

hypothermia an abnormally low body temperature

hypotonicity decreased muscle tone

hypotonic solution a fluid possessing a lesser concentration of solutes than plasma

hypoventilation a reduction in the amount of air entering the lungs, characterized by shallow respirations

hypovolemia decreased blood volume

hypovolemic shock a state of shock due to a reduction in the volume of circulating blood

hypoxemia low partial pressure of oxygen or low saturation of oxyhemoglobin in the arterial blood

hypoxia oxygen deficiency

iatrogenic caused by the physician or medical therapy

ileal conduit method of diverting urinary flow into the ileum

ileostomy an artificial abdominal opening into the ileum (small bowel)

immobility prescribed or unavoidable restriction of movement in any area of a person's life

immunity a specific resistance of the body to infection; it may be naturally endowed resistance or resistance developed after exposure to a disease agent

immunization the process of becoming immune or rendering someone immune

immunoglobulin a part of the body's plasma proteins; also called *immune bodies* or *antibodies*

impaction a condition of being firmly wedged or lodged; in reference to feces, a collection of hardened putty-like feces in the folds of the rectum

incentive spirometer (sustained maximal inspiration device, SMI) a device that measures the flow of air through a mouthpiece as the client practices maximal depth of respiration

incision a cut or wound that is intentionally made, for example, during surgery

incompatibility (of drug) undesired chemical or physical reaction between a drug and an infusion solution, between two or more drugs, or between a drug and the container or tubing

incontinence inability to control the elimination of urine (enuresis) or feces (fecal incontinence)

incubation period the time between the entry of microorganisms into the body and the onset of symptoms of the infection

induration hardening

infarct a localized area of necrosis (dead cells) usually caused by obstructed arterial blood flow to the part

infection the disease process produced by microorganisms

infestation invasion of the body by insects, mites, ticks, and/or parasites

infiltration the diffusion or deposition of substances into a tissue

inflammation local and nonspecific defensive tissue response to injury or destruction of cells

informed consent permission given voluntarily by a mentally competent person for treatment or a special procedure (eg, surgery) that indicates the individual has been provided with information about the treatment and understands it

infusion the introduction of fluid into a vein or part of the body

inhalation (aerosol) therapy delivery of droplets of medication or moisture suspended in a gas, such as oxygen, by inhalation through the nose or mouth

inner canthus the corner of the upper and lower eyelids near the nose

insomnia inability to initiate or maintain a sufficient quality or quantity of sleep

inspection visual examination to detect features perceptible to the eye

instillation application of a medication into a body cavity or orifice

insulin a hormone secreted by the beta cells of the islands of Langerhans in the pancreas; also, a preparation for administration

integument the skin or covering of the body

integumentary system the skin, hair, and nails

intercostal between the ribs

intercostal retractions indrawing between the ribs with respiration

intermittent positive pressure breathing (IPPB) delivery of oxygen into the lungs at positive pressure and release of the pressure passively during expiration

internal rotation a turning toward the midline, such as rotation of the hip joint

interstitial between the cells of the body's tissues

interstitial fluid fluid surrounding the body cells

intestinal distention (tympanites) stretching and inflation of the intestines due to the presence of air or gas

intracellular within a cell or cells

intracellular fluid (cellular fluid, ICF) fluid found within the body cells

intractable pain pain that is resistant to cure or relief

intradermal (intracutaneous) within the skin

intramuscular within or inside muscle tissue

intraoperative period the time during surgery

intrapleural within the pleural cavity

intrapleural pressure pressure within the pleural cavity

intrapulmonic pressure pressure within the lungs

intrathecal within or into the spinal canal

intravascular within a blood vessel

intravenous within a vein

intravenous cholangiogram an x-ray film of the bile ducts after a contrast dye has been administered intravenously

intravenous push (IVP, bolus) direct intravenous administration of a medication that cannot be diluted or that is needed in an emergency

intravenous pyelogram an x-ray film of the kidneys taken after intravenous injection of a radiopaque dye

intravenous pyelography (IVP) x-ray filming of the kidney and ureters after injection of a radiopaque material intravenously; also called *intravenous urography*

intravertebral (intraspinal) within the vertebrae

intubation insertion of a tube

inversion a turning inward

ion an electrolyte

iron deficiency anemia form of anemia caused by an inadequate supply of iron for synthesis of hemoglobin

irradiation exposure to penetrating rays, such as x rays, gamma rays, infrared rays, or ultraviolet rays

irrigation (lavage) the washing of a body cavity or a wound

irritant a substance that stimulates unpleasant responses, that is, irritates

ischemia lack of blood supply to a body part

isolation practice that prevents the spread of infection and communicable diseases

isometric having the same measure or length

isotonic having the same tonicity as the body fluids; the term is used to compare solutions of the same strength or concentration

jaundice a yellowish tinge to the skin and mucous membrane caused by excess bilirubin in the blood

jejunum the portion of the small intestine that extends from the duodenum to the ileum

Kardex a portable card index file that organizes data about clients in a concise way and, often, contains nursing care plans

Kegel's exercises exercises for tightening pelvic floor or perineal muscles

ketosis a condition in which excessive ketones are accumulated in the body

knee-chest position *see* **genupectoral position**

koilonychia an upward curvature of the nail from the nail bed

Korotkoff's sounds a series of five sounds heard when auscultating blood pressure; these sounds are produced by blood within the artery with each ventricular contraction

kyphosis an exaggerated convexity in the thoracic region of the vertebral column, resulting in a stooped posture

labored breathing difficult or dyspneic breathing

lacerate to tear, rather than cut, a body tissue

lacrimal sac the opening connecting the tear ducts in the inner canthus of the eye to the nasolacrimal duct, which empties into the nasal cavity

lacrimation the secretion and discharge of tears

laryngeal stridor a harsh, crowing sound heard during expiration when a laryngeal obstruction is present

laryngoscope a lighted instrument used to visualize the larynx

laryngoscopy visual examination of the larynx with a laryngoscope

laryngospasm spasmodic closure of the larynx

lateral to the side, away from the midline

lateral position a side-lying position

lavage an irrigation or washing of a body organ, such as the stomach

laxative a medication that stimulates bowel activity

lentigo senilis clusters of melanocytes that appear as brown "age" spots

lesion the traumatic or pathologic interruption of a tissue or the loss of function of a body part

lethargy drowsiness; a state in which a person sleeps much of the time when the person is not stimulated

leukocyte a white blood cell

leukocytosis an increase in the number of white blood cells

Levin tube a single-lumen nasogastric tube

ligament a broad, fibrous band that holds two or more bones together

liniment a topical liquid applied to the skin frequently to stimulate circulation or to relieve pain

lithotomy position a back-lying position in which the feet are supported in stirrups

lobar pneumonia an infectious disease of one or more lobes of the lung

lobe a well-defined portion of an organ, for example, of the lung or brain

lordosis an exaggerated concavity in the lumbar region of the vertebral column

louse a parasitic insect that infests mammals (plural: *lice*)

lumbar puncture (LP, spinal tap) the insertion of a needle into the subarachnoid space at the lumbar region

lumen a channel within a tube, such as the channel of an artery in which blood flows

lung compliance expansibility of the lung

lung recoil the tendency of lungs to collapse away from the chest wall

lymph a transparent, slightly yellow fluid found within the lymphatic vessels

lymphadenitis inflammation of the lymph nodes

lymphangitis the inflammation of a lymphatic vessel or vessels

lymphatic referring to lymph or lymph vessels

maceration the wasting away or softening of a solid as if by the action of soaking; often used to describe degenerative changes and eventual disintegration

malaise a general feeling of being unwell or indisposed

malignancy abnormal tissue with a tendency to grow and invade other tissues

malleolus a rounded prominence on the distal end of the tibia or fibula

malnutrition a disorder of nutrition; insufficient nourishment of the body cells

mammography x-ray study of breast tissues

margination the aggregating or lining up of substances along a surface or edge, such as the lining up of white blood cells against the wall of a blood vessel during the inflammatory process

mastectomy surgical removal of the breast

masticate to chew

meatus an opening, passage, or channel

medial toward the middle or midline

medical asepsis practices that limit the number, growth, and spread of microorganisms; clean technique

melanin the dark pigment of the skin

meniscus the crescent-shaped structure of the surface of a column of liquid; the crescent-shaped cartilage in the knee joint

metabolism the sum of all the physical and chemical processes by which living substance is formed and maintained and by which energy is made available for use by the organism

metacarpal referring to the part of the hand between the wrist and fingers

micturate (urinate, void) to pass urine from the body

micturition (urination, voiding) the voluntary expulsion of urine

midclavicular line an imaginary line that runs inferiorly and vertically from the center of the clavicle

midsternal line an imaginary line that runs vertically through the middle of the sternum

miosis constriction of the pupil

MMR combined measles, mumps, and rubella vaccine

mons pubis a pillow of adipose tissue situated over the symphysis pubis and covered by coarse hair; also called the *mons veneris*

Montgomery straps tie tapes used to hold dressings in place

morbidity incidence of disease

mucolytic destroying or dissolving mucus

mucous membrane epithelial tissue that lines passages and cavities communicating with the air

mucus a viscous fluid secreted by the mucous membranes

murmur (cardiac) abnormal sounds heard on auscultation of the heart resulting from turbulent blood flow during systole and diastole

mydriasis enlargement of pupil(s)

mydriatic a medication that dilates the pupils

myelogram an x-ray film of the spinal cord, nerve roots, and vertebrae after injection of a contrast media into the subarachnoid space

myocardial infarction cardiac tissue necrosis resulting from obstruction of the blood flow to the heart

myocardium the heart muscle; the middle layer of the heart tissue

myotonia increased muscle tension or muscle spasm

narcotic antagonist a drug that prevents or reverses the action of a narcotic

nasogastric tube a plastic or rubber tube inserted through the nose into the stomach

nasopharynx the upper part of the pharynx adjoining the nasal passage

natriuresis increased excretion of sodium in the urine

nausea the urge to vomit

nebulizer an atomizer or sprayer

necrosis death of cells or tissue in contact with living cells

necrotic dying

negative nitrogen balance a nitrogen output that exceeds nitrogen intake (related to protein balance)

neoplasm any growth that is new and abnormal

nephritis inflammation of a kidney

nephron the functional unit of the kidney

nephrosis a disease of the kidney in which there is degeneration of kidney function without inflammation; also called *nephrotic syndrome*

nerve block chemical interruption of a nerve pathway effected by injecting a local anesthetic

neurologic pertaining to the nervous system

nocturia (nycturia) increased frequency of urination at night

nocturnal enuresis involuntary urination at night

noncompliance (drug use) failure to follow a prescription

nonproductive cough a dry, harsh cough without secretions

normal saline an isotonic concentration of salt (NaCl) solution

nosocomial referring to or originating in a hospital or similar institution, as in a nosocomial infection

obesity weight that is 20% greater than the ideal for height and frame

objective data client information that can be determined by observation or measurement by laboratory studies or other means and that can be tested against an accepted standard

obturator anything that obstructs or closes an opening; the obturator of a tracheostomy set fits inside and closes off the end of the outer tube

ointment a semisolid preparation applied externally to the body

olfactory referring to the sense of smell

oliguria production of abnormally small amounts of urine by the kidneys

operative (intraoperative) period the time during surgery

ophthalmoscope an instrument used to examine the interior of the eye

opportunistic pathogen microorganism that causes disease only in a susceptible person

orientation awareness of time, place, and person

orifice an external opening of a body cavity; for example, the anus is the orifice of the large intestine

oropharynx the part of the pharynx that lies between the upper aspect of the epiglottis and the soft palate

orthopnea the ability to breathe only in the upright position, that is, sitting or standing

orthopneic position a sitting position in which the client leans over and is supported by an overbed table across the lap

orthostatic hypotension decrease in blood pressure that occurs on assuming a sitting or standing position

osteoarthritis noninflammatory degenerative joint disease

osteomalacia the softening of the bones; decalcification of bones in adults

osteoporosis decrease in bone density; demineralization of bone

ostomy a suffix denoting the formation of an opening or outlet

otoscope an instrument used to inspect the eardrum and external ear canal

outward rotation a turning away from the midline

overweight weight that is 10% greater than the ideal for height and frame

packing filling an open wound or cavity with a material such as gauze

Paco₂ partial pressure of carbon dioxide (arterial blood)

palate the roof of the mouth

palliative affording relief without curing

palliative surgery surgery to relieve the symptoms of a disease process

pallor absence of normal skin color; a whitish-grayish tinge

palpation the act of feeling with the hands, usually the fingers

pandemic an epidemic disease that is widespread

Pao$_2$ partial pressure of oxygen (arterial blood)

papule a small, red, superficial, round elevation of the skin

paracentesis the insertion of a needle into a cavity (usually the abdominal cavity) to remove fluid

paradoxical breathing the ballooning out of the chest wall during expiration and depression or sucking inward of the chest wall during inspiration

paralysis the impairment or loss of motor function of a body part

paraplegia paralysis of the lower part of the body (including the legs) affecting both motor function and sensation

parasites plants or animals that live on or within another living organism

parenchyma the functional or essential elements of an organ

parenteral accomplished by a needle; occurring outside the alimentary tract; injected into the body through some route other than the alimentary canal, for example, intravenously

paresis partial or incomplete paralysis

paresthesia an abnormal sensation of numbness, burning, or prickling

paronychia inflammation of the tissue surrounding the nail

parotitis (parotiditis) inflammation of the parotid salivary gland

passive exercise exercise during which the muscles do not contract and the nurse, therapist, or client supplies the energy to move the client's body part

paste a semisolid dermatologic preparation that is applied externally

patent open, unobstructed, not closed

pathogen a microorganism capable of producing disease

Pco$_2$ partial pressure of carbon dioxide (venous blood)

peak plasma level (of drug) the concentration of a drug in the blood plasma that occurs when the elimination rate equals the rate of absorption

pectoriloquy the clear transmission of vocal sounds through the chest wall during auscultation

pediculosis infestation with lice

penetrating wound a wound created by an instrument that penetrated the skin or mucous membranes deeply into the tissues

Penrose drain a flexible rubber drain

percussion an assessment method in which the body surface is tapped or struck to elicit sound or vibrations from the body structures below the struck area

percutaneous electric stimulation stimulation of major peripheral nerves by electricity applied to the skin surface

perfusion passage of fluid through the vessels of an organ or tissue

perineum the area between the anus and the genitals

perioperative period the time before, during, and after an operation

periorbital around the eye socket

peripheral at the edge or outward boundary

peripheral pulse a pulse located in the periphery of the body

peristalsis wavelike movements produced by circular and longitudinal muscle fibers of the intestinal walls; it propels the intestinal contents onward

peristomal referring to the skin area that surrounds a stoma

peritoneal cavity the area between the layers of peritoneum in the abdomen; a potential space

peritoneum the membrane lining the abdominal walls

peritonitis inflammation of the peritoneum

perspiration the fluid secreted by the sweat glands for excreting waste products and cooling the body

petechiae pinpoint red spots on the skin

pH a measure of the relative alkalinity or acidity of a solution; a measure of the concentration of hydrogen ions

phalanx any bone of the fingers or toes (plural: *phalanges*)

phantom pain pain that remains after the perceived location has been removed, such as pain perceived in a foot after the leg has been amputated

phlebitis inflammation of a vein

phlebothrombosis intravascular clotting with marked inflammation of a vein

phlebotomy opening a vein to remove blood

photosensitive sensitive to light

phrenic referring to the diaphragm

physiotherapist (physical therapist) a member of the health team who provides assistance to clients with musculoskeletal problems

pigeon chest (pectus carinatum) a chest deformity characterized by a narrow transverse diameter, an increased anteroposterior diameter, and a protruding sternum

pinna the external part of the ear

pitch the quality of sound based on the number of vibrations per second or the frequency of vibrations

pitting edema edema in which firm finger pressure on the skin produces an indentation (pit) that remains for several seconds

plantar flexion movement of the ankle so that the toes point downward

plasma the fluid portion of the blood in which the blood cells are suspended

pleural rub (friction rub) a coarse, leathery, or grating sound produced by the rubbing together of the pleura

pneumonia inflammation of the lung tissue

pneumothorax accumulation of air or gas in the pleural cavity

Po₂ partial pressure of oxygen (venous blood)

polydipsia excessive thirst

polyneuritis inflammation of many nerves

polypnea an abnormal increase in the respiratory rate

polyuria (diuresis) the production of abnormally large amounts of urine by the kidneys

popliteal referring to the posterior aspect of the knee

port an opening or entrance

portal an entrance

posterior toward, or at the back of

postoperative (postsurgical) period the time following surgery

postural drainage drainage of secretions from various lung segments by the use of specific positions and gravity

precordium the area of the chest over the heart or lower thorax

preoperative period the time before an operation

prepuce *see* **foreskin**

primary intention healing wound healing that involves minimal or no tissue loss and in which there is minimal granulation tissue and scarring; also referred to as *primary union* or *first intention healing*

proctoscope a lighted instrument used to visualize the interior of the rectum

proctoscopy visualization of the interior of the rectum with a proctoscope

proctosigmoidoscope a lighted instrument used to visualize the rectum and sigmoid colon

proctosigmoidoscopy visual examination of the rectum and sigmoid colon with a proctosigmoidoscope

prodromal period the time from the onset of nonspecific symptoms to the appearance of specific symptoms

prognosis the medical opinion about the outcome of a disease

pronation turning the palm downward; moving the bones of the forearm so that the palm of the hand turns from anterior to posterior in the anatomic position

prone (prone position) lying on the abdomen with the face turned to one side

prophylaxis preventive treatment; prevention of disease

prostatectomy the removal of the prostate gland

prosthesis an artificial part, such as a glass eye, an artificial leg, or dentures

proteinuria the presence of protein in the urine

protocol written plan specifying the procedures to be followed in a particular situation

protraction moving a part of the body forward in a plane parallel to the ground

proximal closest to the point of attachment

pruritus intense itching

ptosis an eyelid that lies at or below the pupil margin; drooping eyelid

ptyalism excessive secretion of saliva

pulmonary embolus a blood clot that has moved to the lungs

pulse the wave of blood within an artery that is created by contraction of the left ventricle of the heart

pulse deficit a difference between the apical and the radial pulses

pulse pressure the difference between the systolic and the diastolic pressures

pulse rate the number of pulse beats per minute

pulse rhythm the pattern of pulse beats and of intervals between beats

pulse volume the force of the blood with each beat produced by contraction of the left ventricle; pulse strength

puncture (stab) wound a wound made by a sharp instrument penetrating the skin and underlying tissues

purulent containing pus

purulent exudate an exudate consisting of leukocytes, liquefied dead tissue debris, and dead and living bacteria

pus a thick liquid associated with inflammation and composed of cells, liquid, microorganisms, and tissue debris

pustule a small elevation of the skin or mucous membrane, or a clogged pore or follicle containing pus

putrid rotten

pyelogram an x-ray film of the kidney and ureter, showing the pelvis of the kidney

pyrexia elevated body temperature; fever

pyuria the presence of pus in the urine

quality (of sound) subjective description of a sound (eg, whistling, gurgling, or snapping)

radial pulse the pulse point located where the radial artery passes over the radius of the arm

radiating pain pain perceived at the source and in surrounding or nearby structures

rales *see* **crackles**

range of motion (ROM) the degree of movement possible for each joint

rebound phenomenon (thermal) the time when the maximum therapeutic effect of a hot or cold application is achieved and the opposite effect begins

reconstitution the technique of adding a solvent to a powdered drug to prepare it for injection

referred pain pain perceived to be in one area but whose source is another area

reflex an involuntary activity in response to a stimulus

reflux backward flow

regeneration the replacement of destroyed tissue cells by cells that are identical or similar in structure and function

regurgitation the spitting up or backward flow of undigested food

rehabilitation the restoration of a person who is ill or injured to the highest possible functional capacity

relapsing fever a fever characterized by periods of normal temperature lasting 1 or more days between periods of fever

remittent fever a fever characterized by a wide range of temperatures, all above normal, over a 24-hour period

renal relating to the kidney

renal dialysis a process in which blood flows from an artery through an artificial membrane that removes impurities; the blood then returns to the client through a vein

renal pelvis the funnel-shaped upper end of each ureter

residual urine the amount of urine remaining in the bladder after a person voids

residual volume (air) the amount of air remaining in the lungs after a person exhales both tidal and expiratory reserve volumes

resonance a low-pitched, hollow sound produced over normal lung tissue when the chest is percussed

respiration the act of breathing; transport of oxygen from the atmosphere to the body cells and transport of carbon dioxide from the cells to the atmosphere

respiratory acidosis (hypercapnia) a state of excess carbon dioxide in the body

respiratory arrest the sudden cessation of breathing

resuscitate to restore life; to revive

retching the involuntary attempt to vomit without producing vomitus

retention (urinary) the accumulation of urine in the bladder and the inability of the bladder to empty itself

retrograde pyelogram an x-ray film taken after a contrast medium is injected through ureteral catheters into the kidneys

retroperitoneal behind the peritoneum

reverse isolation (barrier technique) measures used to prevent certain clients, such as those with severe burns, from coming in contact with microorganisms

reverse Trendelenburg's position a position with the head of the bed raised and the foot lowered, while the bed foundation remains even

Rh factor antigens present on the surface of some people's erythrocytes; persons who possess this factor are referred to as *Rh positive*, whereas those who do not are referred to as *Rh negative*

rhinitis inflammation of the mucous membrane of the nose

rhonchi coarse, dry, wheezy, or whistling sounds, more audible during exhalation as the air moves through tenacious mucus or a constricted bronchus

roentgenogram a film produced by photography with x-rays

rotation turning a bone around its central axis either toward the midline of the body (*internal rotation*) or away from the midline of the body (*external rotation*)

ruga a ridge or fold in the lining of an organ, such as the vagina or the stomach (plural: *rugae*)

Salem sump tube a double-lumen nasogastric tube

sanguineous bloody

sanguineous exudate an exudate containing large amounts of red blood cells

saphenous vein either of two superficial veins of the legs; the greater one extends from the foot to the inguinal region, whereas the lesser one extends from the foot up the back of the leg to the knee joint

scar (cicatric) tissue dense fibrous tissue derived from granulation tissue

sclerosis a process of hardening that occurs from inflammation and disease of the interstitial substance; the term is used to describe hardening of nervous tissues and arterioles

scoliosis a lateral curvature of a part of the vertebral column

sebaceous gland a gland of the dermis that secretes sebum

seborrheic dermatitis a chronic disease of the skin, characterized by scaling and crusted patches on various body areas, such as the scalp

secondary intention healing wound healing that involves the formation of extensive granulation tissue and in which the repair time is lengthy and scarring is extensive

secretion the product of a gland; for example, saliva is the secretion of the salivary glands

sedative an agent that tends to calm or tranquilize

semi-Fowler's position a bed-sitting position in which the head of the bed is elevated at least 30 degrees, with or without knee flexion; also referred to as *low-Fowler's position*

sensitivity quick response, often referring to the response of microorganisms to an antibiotic

septic referring to a disease process produced by microorganisms or to their poisonous products in the blood

serosanguineous composed of serum and blood

serous exudate a watery exudate composed mainly of serum

serum (blood) blood plasma from which the fibrinogen has been separated during clotting

shock acute circulatory failure

sickle-cell anemia a genetic defect of hemoglobin synthesis that accounts for abnormal crescent-shaped erythrocytes; common to Mediterranean and African populations

side effect an unintended action or complication of a drug

sigmoid colon the lower portion of the descending colon of the large intestine

sigmoidoscope a lighted instrument used to examine the sigmoid colon

sigmoidoscopy examination of the interior of the sigmoid colon with a sigmoidoscope

sitz bath (hip bath) bath used to soak a client's pelvic or perineal area

sleep apnea periodic cessation of breathing during sleep

smear material spread across a glass slide in preparation for microscopic study

spasm involuntary contraction of a muscle or muscle group

specific gravity the weight or degree of concentration of a substance compared with the weight of an equal amount of another substance used as a standard; (for example, water used as a standard has a specific gravity of 1, whereas urine in comparison has a specific gravity of 1.010 to 1.025

speculum a funnel-shaped instrument used to widen and examine canals of the body, such as the vagina or nasal canal

sphincter a ringlike muscle that opens or closes a natural orifice (eg, the urethra) when it relaxes or contracts

sphygmomanometer an instrument used to measure the pressure of the blood in the arteries

spirometry the measurement of pulmonary volumes and capacities using a spirometer

splint a rigid bar or appliance used to stabilize a body part

sprain injury of the ligaments and associated structure of a joint by wrenching or twisting; associated structures include tendons, muscles, nerves, and blood vessels

sputum the mucous secretion from the lungs, bronchi, and trachea that is expectorated through the mouth

stasis stagnation or stoppage of flow of body fluids, such as intestinal fluids, urine, or blood

stenosis constriction or narrowing of a body canal, vessel, or opening

sterile free from microorganisms, including spores

sterile field a specified area that is considered free from microorganisms

sterile technique *see* **surgical asepsis**

sterilization a process that destroys all microorganisms, including spores

stertor snoring or sonorous respiration, usually due to a partial obstruction of the upper airway

stethoscope an instrument used to listen to various sounds inside the body, such as the heartbeat

stock supply (of drugs) medications stocked in relatively large quantities on a nursing unit; individual doses are taken from the large supply

stoma an artificial opening in the abdominal wall; it may be permanent or temporary

stomatitis inflammation of the mouth

stool (feces) waste products excreted from the large intestine

stopcock a valve that controls the flow of fluid or air through a tube

strain (of a muscle) overexertion or overstretching of a muscle or part of a muscle

stridor a shrill, harsh, crowing sound made on inhalation; due to constriction of the upper airway or laryngeal obstruction

stroke volume the amount of blood ejected from the heart with each ventricular contraction

stupor a condition of partial or nearly complete unconsciousness; stuporous clients are never fully awakened even when painfully stimulated

stylet a metal or plastic probe inserted into a needle or cannula to render it stiff and to prevent occlusion of the lumen by particles of tissue

subcostal below the ribs

subcutaneous (hypodermic) beneath the layers of the skin

subjective data client information that only the client can give, such as thoughts or feelings

sublingual under the tongue

suborbital beneath the orbit (the bony cavity containing the eyeball)

subscapular below the scapula (shoulder blade)

substernal retractions indrawing beneath the sternum (breastbone)

sudoriferous gland a gland of the dermis that secretes sweat

supination turning the palm upward; moving the bones of the forearm so that the palm of the hand turns from posterior to anterior in the anatomic position

supine (supine position) lying on the back with the face upward; also called *dorsal position*

suppository a solid, cone-shaped, medicated substance inserted into the rectum, vagina, or urethra

supraclavicular retractions indrawing above the clavicles (collarbones)

suprapubic above the pubic arch

suprasternal retractions indrawing above the sternum (breastbone)

surfactant a lipoprotein mixture secreted in the alveoli that reduces surface tension of the fluid lining the alveoli

surgical asepsis measures that render and maintain objects free of all microorganisms including spores (sterile)

suture in surgery, a surgical stitch used to close accidental or surgical wounds; in anatomy, a junction line of the skull bones

symptoms (covert data) *see* **subjective data**

syncope fainting or temporary loss of consciousness

syndrome a group of signs and symptoms resulting from a single cause and constituting a typical clinical picture, such as the shock syndrome

synovial joint a freely movable joint surrounded by a capsule enclosing a cavity that contains a transparent, viscid fluid

syphilis a sexually transmitted disease caused by the microorganism *Treponema pallidum*

syringe an instrument used to inject or withdraw liquids

systemic pertaining to the body (or other system) as a whole

systole the period when the ventricles of the heart are contracted

systolic pressure the pressure of the blood against the arterial walls when the ventricles of the heart contract

tablet a medication in solid form that is compressed and molded

tachycardia an excessively rapid pulse or heart rate, over 100 beats per minute in an adult

tachypnea abnormally fast respirations, usually more than 24 per minute, marked by quick, shallow breaths

tactile (vocal) fremitus vibrations, palpable with the palms of the hands, originating in the larynx and transmitted to the chest wall during speech

T-binder a cloth in the shape of a T often used to retain dressings in the genital region

Td combined tetanus and diphtheria toxoid used for people over 6 years of age; it has less diphtheria toxoid than does DT

temporal pulse a pulse point where the temporal artery passes over the temporal bone of the skull

tenesmus straining; painful, ineffective straining during defecation or urination

tetany a syndrome manifested by muscle twitching, cramps, convulsions, and sharp flexion of the wrist and ankle joints

therapy treatment or remedy

thermography the use of infrared camera to photograph the surface of the body, thus indicating surface temperatures

thoracocentesis insertion of a needle into the pleural cavity for diagnostic or therapeutic purposes

thorax the chest cavity

thrill (cardiac) vibrating sensation indicating turbulent blood flow

thrombocytopenia an abnormal reduction in the number of platelets in the blood

thrombophlebitis inflammation of a vein followed by formation of a blood clot

thrombosis the development of a blood clot

thrombus a solid mass of blood constituents in the circulatory system; a clot (plural: *thrombi*)

tic a repetitive twitching of the muscles, often of the face or upper trunk

tidal volume the volume of air that is normally inhaled and exhaled

tinnitus a ringing or buzzing sensation in the ears

tissue perfusion supplying nutrients and oxygen to body tissues and organs

tomography a scanning procedure during which several x-ray beams pass through the body part from different angles

tonicity the normal condition of tension or tone, for example, of a muscle

tonus the slight, continual contraction of muscles

topical applied externally, for example, to the skin or mucus membranes

tortuous twisted

total lung capacity the maximum volume to which the lungs can be expanded

total parenteral nutrition administration of a hypertonic solution of carbohydrates, amino acids, and lipids by an indwelling intravenous catheter placed into the superior vena cava via the jugular or subclavian vein; also called *intravenous hyperalimentation*

tourniquet a device, such as a rubber strip, that is wrapped around a body area to compress the blood vessels

toxemia a generalized toxic state caused by the distribution of poisonous products of bacteria throughout the body

toxin a poison produced by some microorganisms, animals, and plants

tracheal tug an indrawing and downward pulling of the trachea during inhalation

tracheostomy a procedure by which an opening is made in the anterior portion of the trachea and a cannula is introduced into the opening

traction the exertion of a pulling force

trademark (brand name) name of drug given by the drug manufacturer

transcutaneous electrical nerve stimulation (TENS) the placement of electrodes on the surface of the skin over a peripheral nerve pathway for the purpose of relieving pain

transfusion the introduction of whole blood or its components, such as serum, erythrocytes, or platelets, into the venous circulation

trapeze bar a triangular handgrip suspended from an overbed frame

trauma injury

tremor an involuntary muscle contraction, for example, quivering, twitching, or convulsions

Trendelenburg's position a bed position with the head of the bed lowered and the foot raised, while the bed foundation remains even; in some agencies, the position involves elevation of the knees, with the feet lowered and the head lowered

trocar a sharp, pointed instrument that fits inside a cannula and is used to pierce body cavities

trochanter either of two processes below the neck of the femur

trochanter roll a rolled towel support placed against the hips to prevent external rotation of the legs

troche a lozenge

tumor an uncontrolled and progressive growth of cells

tuning fork an instrument shaped like a two-pronged fork and made of metal; the prongs vibrate when struck

turgor normal cell tension; distention

tympanites (distention) swelling of the abdomen due to the presence of excessive flatus in the intestines or peritoneal cavity

tympany a hollow, drumlike sound produced on percussion over organs that contain gas or air

ulcer a localized sloughing of skin tissue or mucous membrane commonly associated with varicosities or hyperactivity of the gastrointestinal tract

ultrasound high-frequency, mechanical, radiant energy

unconscious incapable of responding to sensory stimuli; insensible

unilateral affecting one side

unit dose system (of drugs) prepackaged and labeled individual doses of medication for each client; the amount of medication the client is to receive at a prescribed hour

universal donor a person with type O blood

universal recipient a person with type AB blood

unsterile containing microorganisms; unsterile material may be clean or contaminated

urea a substance found in urine, blood, and lymph; the main nitrogenous substance in blood

urea frost the appearance of the skin when the salt crystals remain after the evaporation of sweat in urhidrosis

uremia the retention in the blood of excessive amounts of the by-products of protein metabolism

ureteroileosigmoidostomy an artificial opening into the ureters in which the ureters are implanted into the sigmoid colon

ureterostomy an artificial opening into the ureter

urethritis inflammation of the urethra

urgency (urinary) a feeling that one must urinate

urinal a receptacle used to collect urine

urinalysis a laboratory analysis of the urine

urinary diversion *see* **urostomy**

urobilin the oxidized form of urobilinogen, a compound formed from bilirubin, that is found in feces and occasionally in urine

urobilinogen a colorless compound found in the intestines from the reduction of bilirubin

urostomy (ureterostomy, urinary diversion) an opening through the abdominal wall into the urinary tract that permits the drainage of urine

urticaria an allergic reaction marked by smooth, reddened, slightly elevated patches of skin and intense itching

uvula a small fleshy mass projecting from the soft palate above the base of the tongue

vaccine a suspension of killed, attenuated, or living microorganisms administered to prevent or treat an infectious disease

Valsalva maneuver forceful exhalation against a closed glottis, which increases intrathoracic pressure and thus interferes with venous return to the heart

varicosity the state of having swollen, distended, and knotted veins, especially in the legs

vasectomy ligation and cutting of the vas deferens, rendering the male sterile

vasoconstriction a decrease in the caliber (lumen) of blood vessels

vasodilation an increase in the caliber (lumen) of blood vessels

vasopressor an agent that causes the blood pressure to rise

vasospasm spasm or constriction of the blood vessels

ventilation the movement of air; the act of breathing

ventral toward or at the front of; anterior

ventricle a small cavity, such as those located in the brain or the heart

ventriculogram an x-ray film of the ventricles of the brain taken after the introduction of an opaque medium

ventriculography radiologic examination of the ventricles of the brain following the insertion of air or a radiopaque medium

vertigo dizziness

vesicostomy an artificial opening into the bladder in which the anterior wall of the bladder is sutured to the abdominal wall and a stoma is formed from the bladder wall

vesicular sounds normal, quiet, rustling, or swishing respiratory sounds heard over the terminal bronchioles and alveoli during auscultation

vial a glass medication container with a sealed rubber cap, for single or multiple doses

vibration a technique of rapidly agitating the hands while pressing on a body area

virulence the degree of strength or power of an organism to produce disease

virus minute infectious agent smaller than a bacterium

viscera large interior organs in body cavities, such as the liver and stomach (singular: viscus)

visceral referring to viscera

visceral pain pain originating in the viscera

viscosity the quality of being viscous; the thickness or resistance of a fluid

vital capacity maximum amount of air that can be exhaled following a maximum inhalation

vital (cardinal) signs measurement of physiologic functioning—specifically, temperature, pulse, respirations, and blood pressure

vitiligo patches of hypopigmented skin

vocal resonance vibrations of the larynx transmitted during speech through the respiratory system to the chest wall

void urinate, micturate

vomitus material vomited

walker a metal, rectangular frame used as an aid to ambulation

Weber's test a test that assesses bone conduction of sound

wheal *see* **bleb**

wheeze a whistling sound on exhalation that usually indicates narrowing of the bronchial air passages

xiphoid process the tip of the sternum

x rays electromagnetic radiations with extremely short wavelengths

Index